Anouar Jarraya
Manel Kammoun

COVID-19 and pregnancy

Anouar Jarraya
Manel Kammoun

COVID-19 and pregnancy

ScienciaScripts

Imprint
Any brand names and product names mentioned in this book are subject to trademark, brand or patent protection and are trademarks or registered trademarks of their respective holders. The use of brand names, product names, common names, trade names, product descriptions etc. even without a particular marking in this work is in no way to be construed to mean that such names may be regarded as unrestricted in respect of trademark and brand protection legislation and could thus be used by anyone.

Cover image: www.ingimage.com

This book is a translation from the original published under ISBN 978-620-6-71773-7.

Publisher:
Sciencia Scripts
is a trademark of
Dodo Books Indian Ocean Ltd. and OmniScriptum S.R.L publishing group

120 High Road, East Finchley, London, N2 9ED, United Kingdom
Str. Armeneasca 28/1, office 1, Chisinau MD-2012, Republic of Moldova, Europe
Printed at: see last page
ISBN: 978-620-7-92444-8

COVID-19 IN PREGNANCY

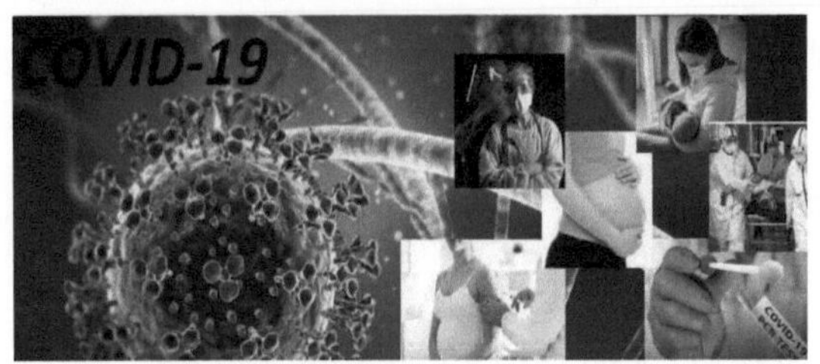

AUTHORS :

MR. ANOUAR JARRAYA DR MALE COMB

TABLE OF CONTENTS

1- INTRODUCTION

COVID-19 is an infectious disease caused by the novel coronavirus SARS-CoV-2 Who East appeared For there first times has Wuhan (China) in December 2019 And Who its propagated quickly In THE world entire And cause a of the more dangerous crises sanitary what has known humanity. This virus has summer has the origin to several waves epidemiological And he n / A not stopped of mutate since he is of an RNA virus thus declaring several strains of varying virulence and contagiousness GOOD that THE SARS-CoV-2 touch all THE slices of ages, what that either gender, it is more serious and can lead to death, especially in fragile situations such as the elderly or those suffering from comorbidities and those suffering from immunosuppression. Pregnant women are also part of this group of fragile people and are known to be vulnerable to viruses in general (1).

Indeed, during pregnancy, women undergo physiological changes which affect the respiratory system through the reduction of pulmonary reserves, associated with a higher oxygen consumption with a edema of the mucous membrane roads respiratory Who could induce a greater morbidity respiratory in case infection of the ways upper respiratory (2). In addition, physiological changes in the immune system cause a decrease in cellular immunity caused by the reduction in effectiveness And of number of the cells of immunity innate (macrophages, Natural killer (NK), cells dendritic) Thus that lymphocytes T (3), This Who could make pregnant women more vulnerable to respiratory viruses or other infections requiring cellular immunity. Particular severity has been reported for the H1N1 influenza virus for example (4,5).

It is important to emphasize that in pregnant women, COVID-19 appears with a wide variety of presentations clinics with a rate not negligible of complications can put in game THE prognosis functional And vital of the patients. Clinical manifestations are generally dominated by fever, cough, gastrointestinal disorders and sometimes by ENT signs.Thus, several complications have been reported such as acute respiratory distress syndrome (ARDS), renal failure, thromboembolic accidents, And Sometimes even of the failures multivisceral Who are likely to impact THE prognosis maternal And fetal (6). These complications are especially more frequent and serious in pregnant women with pregnancy comorbidities Or No gravidic Or having A deficit immune, the infection by SARS-CoV2 can training of the paintings clinics extremely serious responsible of a failure multi-visceral (7). THE stadium of severity of disease And her evolutionary character can to guide there socket in charge And even THE fashion childbirth : Fetal distress due to severe maternal hypoxia or associated severe preeclampsia or labor intolerance should indicate emergency fetal extraction by cesarean section (7). Likewise, emergency cesarean section is considered in the event of maternal rescue in the face of severe ARDS or multiorgan failure, with the aim of improving the woman's adaptation to viral infection (8). Currently, vaginal delivery is strongly recommended by THE companies scholars if THE data clinics And obstetrics are in favor with less of risk worsening kindergarten, All in in holding realize that THE risks of transmission vertical fetal And of reaching of staff of health (9).

HE must Also mention that there disease COVID-19 has evolved with evolution following the mutations experienced by SARS CoV2 which were the cause of increasing contagiousness And of less virulence with THE time. In more, the vaccination anti-COVID-19 has exchange THE demonstrations clinics of there disease Thus that prognosis of affected parturients and maternal-fetal impact. In addition, support is currently well codified.

2- CHANGES PHYSIOLOGICAL AT COURSE OF THERE PREGNANCY AND COVID-19

Pregnant women are considered vulnerable to viral infections and particularly SARS-CoV-2 given the physiological and immunological what undergoes (10). She East characterized by a increased oxygen consumption, explained by increased weight and increased metabolism of base allowing of answer to fetal needs. Else go, lung capacity and oxygen reserves are reduced following changes anatomical reducing mobility of the diaphragm And there chest compliance (8.9). This explain THE risk of desaturation fast And deep in cases of lung damage by the virus (10,11).

In more, on THE plan hemodynamics, there women pregnant knows a increase of there volume increased At 3rd quarter, associated has a anemia of dilution And peripheral vasodilation with capillary hyperpermeability, therefore favoring edema interstitial (12). THE SARS-CoV-2 Who has a affinity For the paths respiratory go train a reaction inflammatory important mediated by a thunderstorm cytokine (a secretion inappropriate of cytokines) Who aims to call the cells of immunity innate (macrophages And polynuclear) towards THE alveoli, which will worsen pulmonary edema and risks destroying the alveolar-capillary barrier, thus leading to ARDS (13,14) (Figure 1).

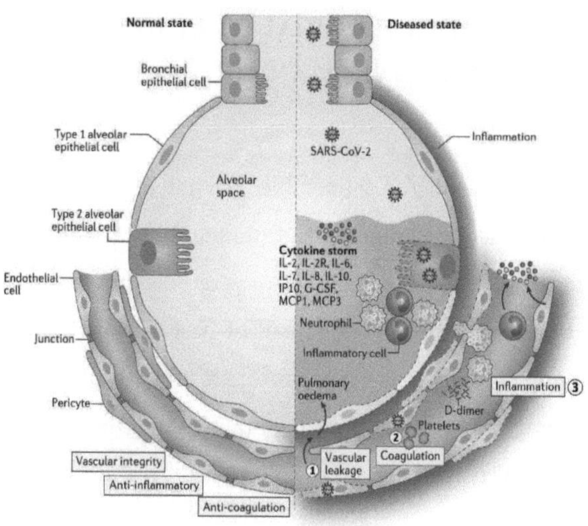

Figure 1: Pathophysiology of ARDS And dysfunction endothelial In COVID-19 (15)

There reaction inflammatory intense go enable in more THE cells endothelial cells of the pulmonary capillaries, which further promotes the passage of fluid and immune cells towards the alveolus with the release of postman tissue by endothelial cells can activate platelet aggregation. This reaction adds to the pro-coagulant effect of interleukin 6, which could trigger a process of thrombosis in these capillaries in a field known for its hypercoagulability (increased synthesis of factors and inhibition fibrinolysis) and by blood stasis which thus expose the pregnant woman to an additional risk of thromboembolic accidents (15,16) (Figure 2).

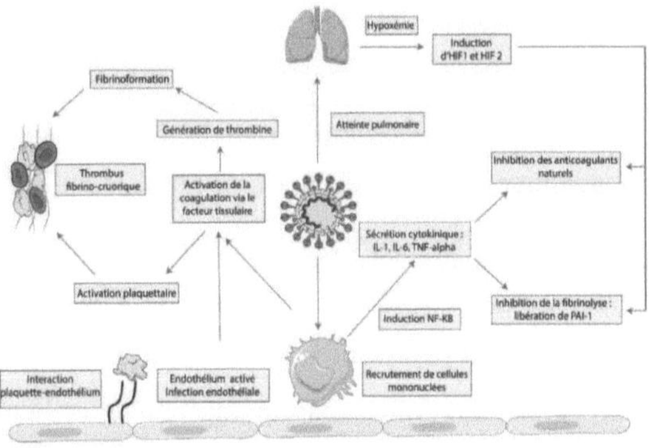

Figure 2 : THE mechanisms of there coagulopathy linked has there COVID-19 (16)

In consideration, THE placenta, Who East the interface exchange between there mother And THE fetus, presents the receptors for angiotensin converting enzyme-2 (ACE-2) target of the S protein of SARS-CoV-2, which argues in favor of the risk of vertical transmission and also in favor of the risk of placental infection and endothelial dysfunction affecting the placental vasculature (15) (Figure 3). By THE same mechanisms, he exist A risk of microthrombi leading has placental ischemia causing fetal distress and "preeclampsia-like syndrome" (15,16, 17).

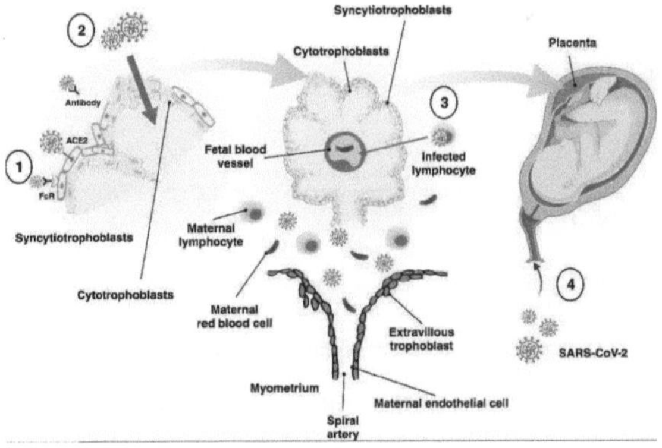

Figure 3 : Mechanisms And risks of there transmission vertical (15)

On THE plan immune, For adapt has there graft semi-allogeneic that constitutes the fetus, the immune system experiences modifications of innate immunity, playing the role of antigen-presenting cells essential for differentiation of the cells of immunity adaptive, by there decrease of number and of there ability of phagocytosis of the macrophages, of the cells dendritic And NKs. Immunity cellular East also touched following has A imbalance between T helper 1 and 2 (Th1/Th2) lymphocytes. This particular immune profile, in which helper 2 type cytokines predominate, will favor humoral immunity over cellular immunity and will result in an inability to eliminate infected cells due to the lack of cytotoxic T lymphocytes. However, the answer of wife pregnant to vaccination is respected because the production antibodies by plasma cells, originating from B lymphocytes differentiated under the effect of the cytokines of the Th2, East maintained And THE passage of these antibody has through THE placenta East NOW confirmed (18). This immunity acquired passively speak new born could THE protect during a few month After her birth (19).

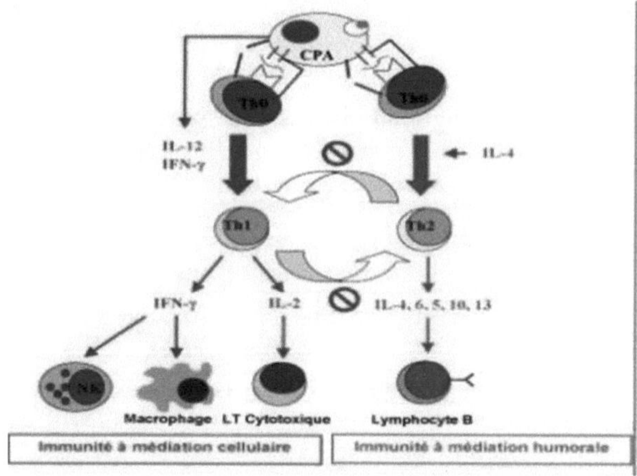

Figure 4 : Achievement of immunity cellular at the house of there women pregnant and impact on COVID-19

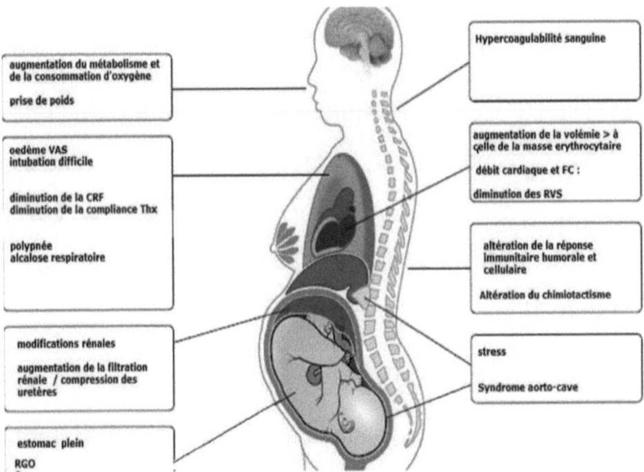

Figure 5 : Changes physiological At course of there pregnancy And COVID -19

SARS CoV2 is characterized by its spike protein (Prot S) which has the ability to recognize the ACE receptor on the surface of the host cell. The passage of the virus inside the cell occurs via facilitator proteins such as TMPRSS2. This passage East OBLIGATORY For there replication viral And there manifestation of the disease (figure 4).

Since its appearance, SARS-CoV2 has continued to mutate. It is in fact a virus has RNA Who se characterizes by of the errors during of there replication viral which is done via the host cell's machine. These mutations were at the origin of the different variants of virus Who have summer has the origin of the different waves Who hit the world (Figure 5).

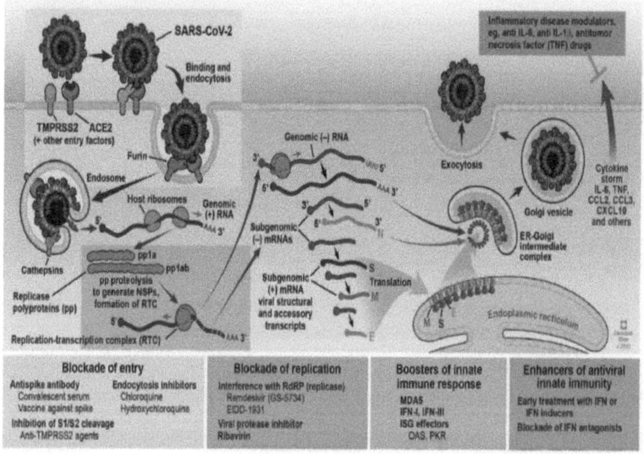

Figure 6 : replication viral of SARS CoV2 And diversion of there host cell machine. (20)

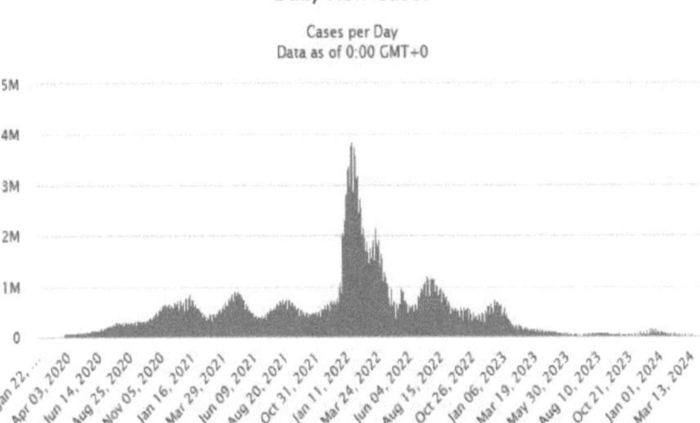

Figure 7 : evolution of there COVID-19 in waves

(https://www.worldometers.info/coronavirus)

Several variants have summer announced : alpha (B.1.1.7), Beta (B.1.351), Gamma (P.1), Delta (B.1.617.2), and finally the Omicron (B.1.1.529). These variants have pathogenicity (virulence) and contagiousness different and very variable. Moreover, the Omicron variant of SARS-CoV-2 (B.1.1.529), detected for the first time in November 2021, characterized by A power of contagion without previous. This Who has do of her there variant there more widespread in the world some months After her appearance, exceeding from afar the variants previous ones such that there variant Delta (B.1.617.2) (21,22). But it appears to cause a less severe acute illness with a low risk of progression in Syndrome of Distress Respiratory Acute (ARDS) by report to other previous strains, at least in vaccinated populations (21). Currently, some believe that this strain called "Omicron" indicates the end of the pandemic even though COVID-19 will persist (21). In front there big virulence And THE rate of death very important In the wave delta which presented the peak of the disease where the health system was overwhelmed in several countries of the world, the authors consider 3 phases of the disease (table 1)

waves pre- delta -alpha. (B.1.1.7) - Beta. (B.1.351) - Gamma (P.1)	Low contagion favored by confinement and panic of there disease promoting use of the means of individual protection and isolation of affected patients but a heavy mortality Above all at the house of THE women speakers.
There delta wave Delta. (B.1.617.2)	Se characterizes by THE peak of there disease with exacerbation of the number of cases while vaccination is not yet generalized Above all In THE country in course of development
Waves post- Delta " Omicron » (B.1.1.529)	These waves are characterized by a reduction in severe forms and the number of hospitalizations which could be linked to the generalization of vaccination and the appearance of passive immunization in the population. No vaccinated but Who has had A contact with THE variants previous ones.

Painting 1 : features of the waves of there COVID-19 at the house of there

pregnant woman

However, caution should be exercised regarding the impact of this new variant on of the patients has high risk, such that THE women speakers (23), And this despite the role of vaccination in reducing the severity of clinical forms. And the prognosis of the disease. It is also prudent to take into consideration the effectiveness of vaccines on this variant characterized by a high risk of vaccine escape or immune evasion (22).

4- DEMONSTRATIONS CLINICS OF THERE COVID-19 AT THE HOUSE OF THERE WOMEN PREGNANT

At beginning of the pandemic, of many questions se are asked about the effects of COVID-19 on pregnant women, especially if the pregnancy increases there sensitivity has the infection by THE SARS-CoV-2, if THE women pregnant women were more likely to have severe illness and if SARS-CoV-2 infection increased THE risk of issues unfavorable For there pregnancy. He y had also a lot of discussions which focus on the mode of delivery if it is conditioned by there severity of there disease And THE role of fashion delivery to prevent transmission of the virus. In this context, the series of literature describing THE results maternal And fetal has there following of this infection, have showed very varied and even biased results because the means offered for support and access to care could vary from one country to another without taking into consideration the notion of different variants of SARS-CoV-2, having a power to contagion and variable virulence (24). From where comes the necessity of describe the characteristics clinics, organic And radiological of there COVID-19 at the house of of pregnant women taking into account the country and the wave, to look for risk factors for severe forms and to assess maternal morbidity and mortality. Studies that focus on both maternal and fetal data are more present in the literature and contribute to enriching knowledge has This subject And present A bring considerable For there practical. In addition, the search for risk factors for severe forms remain essential and have a great clinical impact, especially on informing patients about the prognosis and taking precautions during treatment such as reserving a place in intensive care. Symptoms reported in the event of COVID-19 infection in a woman pregnant is not not different of that described in out of there pregnancy. The big one majority of the women born would feel that of light symptoms of rhinitis or A flu syndrome banal with potentially of the cough, more rarely a fever or dyspnea. The triad of cough, fever and dyspnea is very suggestive of COVID-19. Zohra S Lassi et al (24), carried out a systematic review of the literature and a meta-analysis on 31,016 pregnant women affected by COVID-19. The 62 included studies came from 44 countries belonging to 6 continents, while that close of there half (42.5%) of the case were asymptomatic. The most reported symptoms were cough (51.5%), fever (44.1%), asthenia (26.7%) and anosmia/ageusia (25.1%). Other common symptoms reported included there dyspnea (24.1%), myalgia (20.7%), sore throat (18.1%) and nausea/vomiting (14.2%). This could be explained by the degree of screening and availability of means to carry out this screening.

Sarah Nilkece And al (25), have made a other review systematic literature and a meta-analysis including 34 items with 412 women infected pregnant women by SARS-CoV-2. The most common signs and symptoms were fever (49.7%), dyspnea (31.5%), cough (26.5%), asthenia (8.2%), myalgia (7. 0%), there diarrhea (4.8%) And odynophagia (3.6%). THE biological results most currents were : elevation of there CRP (37.8%), lymphopenia (20.3%), leukopenia (14.2%) and neutrophilia (5.5%).Concerning the radiological results by CT scan or chest X-ray, 51.4% of pregnant women presented a characteristic ground-glass image of viral pneumonia and 51.5% had bilateral lung involvement. (25). In our series, the recourse to to scan thoracic was limited to patients with severe forms or in whom pulmonary embolism is suspected, This Who explain THE rate less important of explorations especially in pregnant women. Jianhua Chi et al (26), carried out a systematic review of the literature and a meta-analysis summarizing the clinical characteristics and maternal-fetal outcomes. This study included 230 pregnant women. The most common symptoms among them were fever (59.05%) and cough (54.76%). Myalgia, shortness of breath, headache and diarrhea were observed in 12.75%, 11.90%, 11.35% and 5.06% patients, respectively. For biological examinations, 40.71% of patients developed lymphopenia. The platelet count showed thrombocytopenia in 4.03% pregnant women. Plasma concentrations of transaminases, CRP and D-Dimers were respectively elevated in 25%, 64.34% and 82.14% of patients.A other review systematic of there literature And a meta-analysis done by Farida Elshafeey And al (27), has identified 33 studies original including 385 women affected by there COVID-19 during there pregnancy and or childbirth. Of the symptoms At moment of diagnostic have summer reported at the house of there mostly of the women (92.5%). Let us note that THE symptoms THE more frequent were : there fever (67.3%), the cough (65.7%), there dyspnea (7.3%), there diarrhea (7.3%), THE ailments of throat (7.0%), asthenia (7.0%) and myalgia (6.2%). Other symptoms were reported in less than 5% of the women who included congestion nasal, rash, THE sputum productive, THE ailments of head, THE discomfort and the loss appetite. So, THE results organic included a elevation of the D-Dimers in 22.3% of cases, elevation of CRP in 18.7% of cases, lymphopenia in 14.0%, slight increase in liver enzymes (AST (5.7%), ALAT (5.45%)) And a thrombocytopenia at the house of 1.0% of the women. Chest imaging was performed in 41.8% of women. But usable data was only available for 32.5% of cases. Typical chest CT features were observed bilaterally in 79.2% of women and unilaterally in 17.6%. No abnormalities on chest CT were reported in 3.2% of women (63). It is sometimes remarkable that there is of the variations of the signs clinics of the disease of a series has the other. This must be interpreted according to the period of the study because the virus has undergone mutations and has given several variants having of the symptoms different (6), that could be due to patient selection, where some studies included asymptomatic forms that did not require hospitalization. He is clear that the clinical manifestations of the disease vary in severity from one subject has A other And this could be explain by THE Status immune And can be genetic factors or the viral load during contamination but certainly the different paintings of severities will allow us of stratify the severity of the disease. Objective criteria may be useful except that it should be noted that the symptomatology has an evolving aspect, particularly in pregnant women who can have a rapid deterioration in their clinical condition and can go from a minor form to a critical form in a short time. of time which requires continuous monitoring and evaluation of the clinical condition of parturients.

It should also be mentioned that there is no timeline for the onset of symptoms or for evolution over time because certain forms of the disease manifest directly through complications. Thromboembolic complications present a reason for the appearance of the disease with phlebitis in the lower limbs, pulmonary embolisms sometimes immediately massive or even cerebral thrombophlebitis. The incidence of these thromboembolic accidents was more marked during the Delta wave. Let's remember Also that there preeclampsia maybe A symptom of there COVID-19 which can cause thrombosis in the villous circulation and lead to ischemia placental. Other neurological complications such as Guillain Barre have summer associated has there COVID-19 Above all during of there wave " Omicron » (23).

	Groupe « Delta » n= 84	Groupe « Omicron » n= 45	Valeur de p
Asymptomatiques (%)	3 (3.5%)	10 (22.2%)	0.001
Toux	64 (76.1%)	27 (60%)	0.032
Fièvre	58 (69%)	17 (37.7%)	0.001
Maux de tête et asthénie	51 (60.7%)	25 (55.5%)	0.314
Dyspnée	31 (36.9%)	7 (15.5%)	0.021
Signes Digestifs (nausée, Vomissements, diarrhée..)	18 (21.4%)	6 (13.3%)	0.208
Autres (maux de gorge , Rhinorrhée , anosmie et Agueusie)	9 (10.7%)	2 (4.4%)	0.194
Pré-éclampsie	18 (21.4%)	12 (26.6%)	0.375
Anémie	11 (13%)	11 (24.4%)	0.133
Cytolyse	11 (13%)	7 (15.5%)	0.419
Thrombopénie < 50000	0 (0%)	1 (2.2%)	0.176
Signes radiologiques > 50% (oui/non)	7/5	3/0	0.266
Besoin en O2 < 6L/min	37 (78.7%)	13 (86.6%)	0.008
Besoin en O2 > 6L/min	7 (14.9%)	0	0.233
Besoin en O2 > 15L/min Techniques avancées (Optiflow ou CPAP)	3 (6.4%)	2 (13.4%)	-
Admission en unité de soins intensifs	2 (2.3%)	3 (6.6%)	0.230

Painting 2: comparison between there variant delta And Omicron At during pregnancy (21):

Shapes clinics	Definition
Asymptomatic	- PCR Or test fast positive without none sign clinical
Shape minor	Not pneumonia Cough dried light Faintness, headaches, pain muscular Signs ENT : pharyngitis Anosmia, ageusia, not dyspnea
Shape moderate	- Pneumonia without sign of severity - Cough, embarrassed respiratory - FR < 30 cpm - SpO2 ≥ 94%
Shape severe	Dyspnea FR ≥ 30 cpm And or SpO2 < 94% has the air ambient
Shape critical	Distress vital, State of shock, sepsis All failure of organs Need for invasive or non-invasive respiratory assistance .

Painting 3 : Classification of the shapes clinics

AA: air ambient; SpO2 : saturation pulsed in oxygen; FR : frequency respiratory; cpm: cycles per minute; The evaluation of there severity of there disease East basically clinical. However, other biological and radiological factors may be taken into account. consideration. It appears that age > 35 years, BMI > 30 mg/m2, preeclampsia, delay in taking in charge And hospitalization, there dyspnea, there cytolysis And the attack pulmonary > 50% on chest CT were identified as risk factors for severe COVID-19 during pregnancy (22). In some studies, pulmonary and other pre-existing comorbidities (hypertension and diabetes) were the main risk factors in pregnant women and the general population.Manon Vouga And al (28), have accomplished a study prospective investigating THE maternal outcomes and risk factors for severe forms in pregnant women affected of there COVID-19. This study has included 1079 parturients. In a multivariate analysis adjusting for risk factors for COVID-

19 severity, pulmonary comorbidities, hypertensive disorders, and diabetes were significantly associated with an increased risk of serious maternal outcomes. A meta-analysis recent done by John Allotey And al. including 435 studies showed that the increase of age maternal, BMI pupil And there preeclampsia were associates has a COVID-19 severe At course of there pregnancy, This which was comparable to our results (29).

Celso Tutiya et al, carried out a single-center study including 114 women. Age gestational At moment of diagnostic > 35 HER, age maternal > 34 years have also been reported as risk factors for severity (30). It seems that THE 3rd quarter of pregnancy present A criteria of severity related to physiological changes accentuated at the end of pregnancy.

In besides, We have observed that THE deadline between THE beginning of the symptoms and hospitalization was A postman of gravity. This setting reflects there difficulty accessing hospitals in developing countries during COVID-19 waves. A study carried out by Mariane O Menezes et al in Brazil, showed that ethnicity black, alive in area peri-urban, without none access At system of care of health of country, Or alive has more of 100 kilometers of the hospital, was associated with increased risk of maternal morbidity and poor prognosis (31). Similar results have been reported in the United States and Great Britain where categories social THE more destitute were victims of the shapes THE more severe illness due to difficulties in accessing care and self - medication (32,33). Yanyan Wu et al (34), carried out a meta-analysis including 45 studies, which showed that patients suffering from severe forms had a significantly higher incidence of abnormal transaminases on admission compared to women with moderate and paucisymptomatic. A achievement pulmonary of > 50% se present as A postman predictive side effects serious. THE role of there CT scan For assess of the lung damage and prediction of severe forms has already been reported in some studies. The extent of the lesions was correlated with the risk of hypoxemia, by direct attack of the exchanger during of the ARDS, Who East involved In there physiopathology of multiorgan failures observed during COVID-19 (35,36,37). The most recent and broad meta-analysis, recently published by Smith, including the data of 21977 patients of 33 country, find that at the house of THE women speakers with A SARS-CoV-2, A GOLD has 2.13 (I.C. 95 % : 1.53–2.95) For THE admission rate in unit of care intensive, has 2.59 (I.C. 95 % : 2.28–2.94) For invasive ventilation and 2.02 (95% CI 1.22–3.34) for ECMO compared to women No pregnant with there Covid-19. In comparing Next to uninfected pregnant women, the death rate was increased with an OR of 2.85 (I.C. 95 % : 1.08–7.52), THE rate of transfer unit of care intensive also with an OR of 18.58 (95% CI: 7.53–45.92) and there were more premature deliveries with an OR of 1.47 (95% CI: 1.14–1.91) (38)

- Age de la parturiente > 35 ans
- Comorbidités : obésité, HTA, Diabète
- 3ème trimestre de grossesse et le péri partum
- Accouchement par césarienne
- Facteurs génétiques
- Accès au soins limité (catégories sociales pauvres et ditance par rapport à l'hopital > 100 Km) et Automédication
- Formes cliniques sévères avec défaillance multi-viscérale
- La variante Delta par rapport à l'Omicron
- Perturbations biologiques (Troubles ionique, insuffisance rénale, cytolyse croissante, D-Dimères très élevés)
- TDM : étendue de la pneumonie > 50%.

Painting 4 : Recapitulation on THE Factors of risks For THE severe forms of COVID-19 during pregnancy

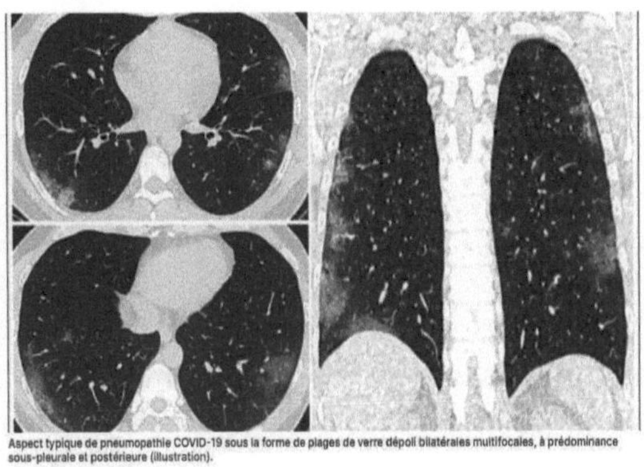

Figure 8 : Appearance radiological of there COVID -19.

5- MORBI-MORTALITY KINDERGARTEN AND FETAL LINKED HAS THERE COVID -19

5.1. Complications specific of there pregnancy : there preeclampsia

There occurrence of there COVID-19 At course of there pregnancy amplified THE role of the factors involved In THE development of the shapes severe of orders hypertensive of pregnancy. SARS-CoV-2 virus causes renin angiotensin system dysfunction and vasoconstriction in attaching to the AT2 receptor of the ACE. Its endothelial tropism simultaneously increases the endothelial dysfunction of the syndrome. THE serum of the women pregnant, having summer infected by THE SARS-CoV-2, but without preeclampsia, contains of the rate students of sFlt-1 And of PlGF. Finally, the significant inflammatory syndrome of COVID-19 increases that involved in severe forms of hypertensive disorders of pregnancy (38). An Italian study has compared THE rate of sFlt-1 And THE report sFlt-1/PlGF (marker pen of oxidative stress of syncytiotrophoblast And of endothelium) women pregnant with and without hypertensive disorders, with and without SARS-CoV-2 infection. The sFlt-1/PlGF ratio is elevated in women with hypertensive disorders of pregnancy, whether they were infected (n = 19) or not (n = 185). The prevalence of orders hypertensive East, in revenge, more high at the house of THE women infected (34% vs 5–8%) (39). The placental lesions observed following pregnancies complicated by COVID-19 confirm the impact of the infection on the placental vascularization. Criteria for poor placental perfusion are also found in the majority of the case of shapes severe of COVID-19 happened during there pregnancy, with a frequency much higher than that observed in a large control population free from COVID-19 (40). in a large meta-analysis, constructed from of 40 studies, documents mortality neonatal increased of almost a third (OR = 1.28) and maternal mortality of almost 40% (OR = 1.37) (41). Among the factors associated with this increased risk, hypertensive disorders of pregnancy were quickly recognized. On the one hand, the presence of cardiovascular risk factors, excess weight, diabetes, hypertension arterial, worsen THE prognosis of the infection by SARS-CoV-2, including during pregnancy, but, on the other hand, these hypertensive disorders of pregnancy are more frequent when the infection occurred during gestation, affecting 20 to 34% of women (42,43).

There shape severe represented by there preeclampsia East also more frequent during pregnancy complicated by COVID-19, with an increased risk in varying proportions depending on the studies (from 20% to 200%), but constant (44,45) . In a Tunisian series, 38 cases (18.90%) of hypertensive pathologies were noted; testifying to the high frequency of this complication in the event of an association of there pregnancy with the infection COVID In OUR population North African (46).

5.2. Mortality kindergarten :

In our context, we noted 7.46% maternal mortality in peripartum in pregnant women with COVID-19 (46). Our results are comparable to international data. (Table XXII) This rate greatly exceeds the maternal mortality rate, in Tunisia estimated at 44 per 100,000 births. alive, This Who testifies that THE SARS-COV-2 East A postman of risk of mortality kindergarten. To UNITED STATES, At course of the year 2021, 1205 women died of maternal causes during pregnancy or within 42 days of giving birth. This number was 861 in 2020 and 754 in 2019, indicates a study of National Center of statistics on there health. In 2021, THE rate mortality has reached 32.9 death For 100 000 births, in comparison of 23.8 per 100,000 in 2020, from 20.1 for 100,000 in 2019 and 17.4 per 100,000 in 2018 (47) This is the highest maternal mortality rate in industrialized countries (24).

Initial CDC data that emerged in 2021 indicated that if pregnant patients were more susceptible of require a admission in ICU Or a mechanical ventilation than their age-matched non-pregnant pairs, their risk of death was not significantly different. Sixteen deaths (0.2%) linked to COVID-19 have summer reported at the house of of the women pregnant elderly of 15 has 44 years, and 208 (0.2%) of these deaths were reported in non-pregnant women (RR: 0.9, 95% CI: 0.5-1.5) (48). However, an updated report from the Centers for control And there prevention of the diseases extending until october 2022 has revealed that in more of the women pregnant requiring more frequently a admission taking care intensive, he y had A risk increased of 70 % of death at the house of THE pregnant women by report to women No pregnant affected of COVID-19 (RR : 1.7, CI has 95 % : 1.2 -2.4) (49). There date of occurrence of death maternal East In the majority of the case in post parturition at the house of THE patients COVID positive (67). This is explained by there severity of painting COVID, Who imposed a extraction fetal emergency for maternal and/or fetal rescue (50) THE complications specific of the infection by SARS-CoV-2 were THE more frequently incriminated with a variable frequency between 38 and 86% for ARDS, between 17 and 39% for septic shock and between 2 and 14% for complications there preeclampsia (51,52). The hemorrhage of post parturition, despite its increased incidence in COVID-positive women, was not associated with increased maternal mortality (53).

5.3. Morbidity fetal And neonatal

- There suffering fetal

Concerning abnormalities in the recording of the fetal heart rate (FHR) in outside the work, literature is sparsely provided. We identified only one study, that of Kahankova. In this cohort of 262 full-term pregnancies noted a rate of 4% anomalies of RCF in out of work at the house of THE women suffering from COVID against a rate 1.5% in unaffected patients. This rate drops to 1.6% for infected and asymptomatic patients. The most observed anomalies were there fetal tachycardia (52%) And RCF micro-oscillating (31%) (53).

- Delay of growth intrauterine

The infection At 3rd quarter n / A none impact on there fetal growth, what regardless of the virus variant and the severity of the clinical picture (54). On the other hand, the infection At 2nd quarter can be responsible of a IUGR in END of pregnancy. This growth delay is generally moderate and has no impact on subsequent neonatal prognosis (55). In our series (46), we identified 13 cases of IUGR (3.49%), the vascular origin was the etiology in all cases.

		Effectif	Pourcentage
RCIU	< 3ème percentile	4	2%
	3-10ème percentile	9	1.49%
Anomalies doppler ombilical	Résistances élevées	5	2.48%
	Diastole nulle	1	0.49%
Anomalies doppler cérébral		2	1%
Anomalies du liquide amniotique	Oligoamnios	6	1.49%
	Hydramnios	2	1%
Anomalies de l'ERCF	Tachycardie	12	4.47%
	Micro-oscillations	14	6.96%
	Décélérations	6	2.98%

Painting 5 : THE data of ultrasound obstetric (46)

- Prematurity

The prematurity rate in our population is relatively high at 27.36%. HAS This day, the bigger source of morbidity And mortality potential For newborns of mothers infected by THE COVID seems be A rate increased childbirth premature, in particular childbirth premature iatrogenic in the context of a serious maternal infection. He exist of the evidence that there COVID-19 increase THE risk childbirth premature. A case study conducted early in the pandemic with 116 pregnant women ruled out the possibility of premature or with individuals infected with SARS-CoV-2, However that contrast with others reports more recent (56). THE data collected with of people (not = 342 080) Who have given birth between May 2020 and January 2021 in England reported that those who underwent infection by THE SARS-CoV-2 (not = 3 527) had a impact more high incidence of adverse pregnancy outcomes, including premature birth (57). That East in correlation with a vast study of cohort on 759 people Swedish Who has clearly noted A risk more pupil childbirth premature in pregnancies affected by COVID-19 (58).

In the United States, 2020 COVID-NET data showed a higher prevalence (nearly 12.6%) of preterm birth among pregnant women with COVID-19 compared to the general population in 2018 (10.0 %). From these data, symptomatic individuals also showed an increased risk (23.1%) of preterm birth (59). And in accordance has these reports, a review systematic watch that THE rate Reported preterm births in COVID-19 patients vary widely between studies, ranging from 14.3% to 61.2% (60). Despite there variety of the reports clinics available, he exist A certain consensus between them on the fact that there is a link close relationship between premature birth and symptomatic COVID-19 during pregnancy. This increase, interested also THE childbirth premature iatrogenic as shown in a national study carried out in the United Kingdom (61).However, outside of cases of induced prematurity, these reports raise unanswered questions about the underlying mechanisms that may lead to premature birth during SARS-CoV-2 infections. For example, there is of the evidence of a small study Who watch that THE cells immune expressing ACE2 are capable to infiltrate THE placenta, This Who can Again aggravate SARS-CoV-2 infection and increase the risk of premature deliveries as well as placental infection (62).

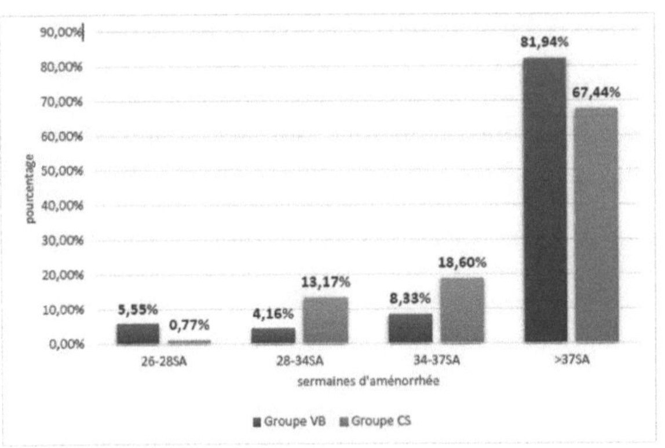

Figure 9 : Term of there pregnancy At moment of childbirth (46)

- **Transmission vertical**

We collected 5 cases of vertical transmission (2.48%) by performing RTPCR in newborns born to mothers infected with COVID-19 at the time of delivery (46). However, this value is far from being representative, of do of the absence of a exam of diagnostic systematic for everyone THE newborns from of women COVID positive. There contamination fetal via the transplacental route seems exceptional. This is linked to the fact that outside of shapes serious, there viremia East weak And transient In there COVID, found in only 1% of symptomatic people, as in most respiratory infections (63). The few neonatal infections reported most likely corresponded to postnatal rather than transplacental contamination. Some studies showed there presence antibodies in the cord blood . In the majority of cases, these were maternal IgG type antibodies, which have the ability to cross the placenta. In a few cases, IgM was found, they would be original fetal because THE IgM kindergarten born do not cross the placenta, however the specificity of these antibodies remains to be clarified despite It is an argument in favor of there possibility of there transmission vertical especially since rare cases of SARS CoV2 placentitis have been identified in more than the cells trophoblastic present THE receiver ACE2 Who East there target of virus (64). A French study reported a neonatal infection in a woman with an infection symptomatic at 35SA, with transmission vertical demonstrated by the presence of viruses in the amniotic fluid (65). Maternal-fetal contamination is therefore possible but probably exceptional (less than 1%).Definitive proof of transplacental transmission of SARS-CoV-2 will require carefully designed studies with appropriate control measures and inclusion/exclusion criteria, in addition to in vivo experimental work that goes beyond observational reports . Future studies should also seek to understand the extent of natural passive immunity conferred by the COVID-19-infected mother to the fetus.

6- PREVENTION OF THERE TRANSMISSION OF THERE COVID-19

THE SARS CoV2 East A virus Who se transmit basically by way respiratory. This is why wearing a mask is an essential step for prevention. The simple surgical mask could reduce the risk of contamination. However, the FFP2 mask helps prevent this risk is 95%. In the more the virus can be transmitted by handling seen that the virus can survive on THE surfaces And exist In THE secretions of the patients (urine, stools, ..etc). Hand hygiene could prevent this risk. Isolation measures must also be taken into account. For affected subjects because their implementation Quarantine for 5 to 10 days following infection helps reduce their contact and prevent the spread of the disease to other patients. These measures are also applicable for pregnant women except that specific protocols must be established For THE women affected by THE SARS CoV2 And Who wish breastfeed their babies. Please note that breast milk does not contain the virus and amniotic fluid In of the case exceptional, This Who do that breastfeeding maternal can be carried out subject to good hygiene and disinfection of skin and surfaces of contact And THE port of mask by there mother And he must Also opt For an airy room. For THE staff of there health, he exist of the protocol hygiene more strict with wearing an FFP2 mask, face protection, and wearing gowns. In addition, the strict application of COVID-19 patient circuits and waste circuits established in the obstetric unit is mandatory in order to avoid contamination of unaffected patients. It should also be remembered that nursing staff must have and validate the necessary training for wearing and removing this equipment. in order to to avoid of the mistakes Who could be source of contamination.

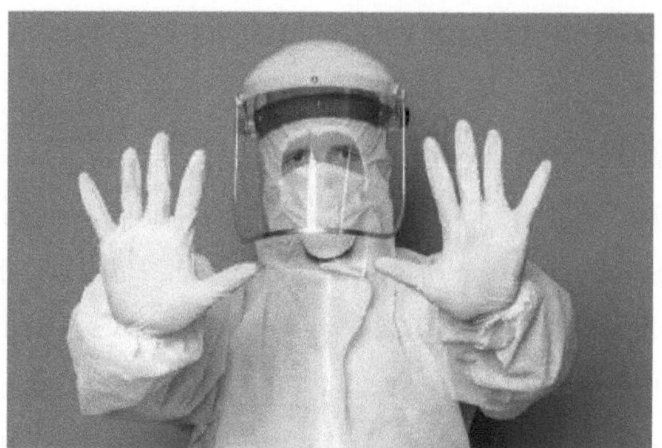

Figure 10 : equipment of protection individual of staff of there health

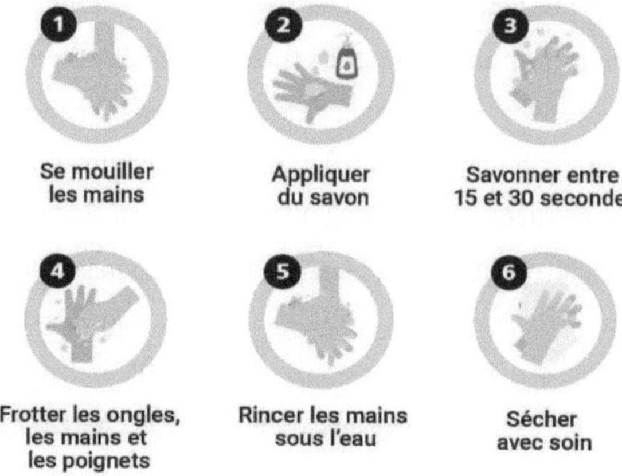

Figure 11 : hygiene hands

7- SOCKET IN CHARGE OF THERE COVID-19 AT THE HOUSE OF THERE WOMEN PREGNANT

7.1. THE treatment symptomatic

The treatment will essentially depend of the severity of painting clinical as mentioned in the following table:

Shapes clinics	Socket in charge
Asymptomatic	- Paracetamol
Shape minor	Treatments symptomatic Not hospitalization Vitamin therapy (Lives VS, D, Zinc)
Shape moderate	Treatment symptomatic Anticoagulation prophylactic if hospitalization or TE risk: 14 days monitoring daily
Shape severe	Treatment symptomatic Oxygen therapy (SpO2>94%) Corticotherapy Anticoagulation prophylactic Or curative antibiotic therapy if superinfection
Shape critical	Transfer in resuscitation Oxygen therapy by MHC, OHD, NIV Or VMI. Corticotherapy Anticoagulation Antibiotic therapy if infections

Painting 6 : Principles of there socket in charge according to there gravity symptoms

MHC : mask has high concentration, OHD : oxygen therapy has high debit,

NAV: ventilation No invasive ; VMI : ventilation invasive mechanics

Telescope oxygen 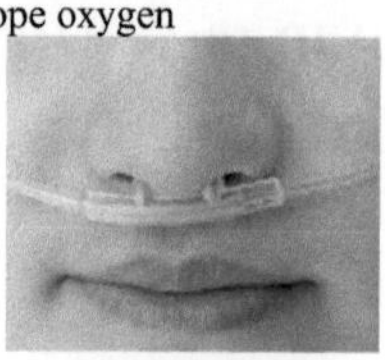	Respiratory support with high FiO2 flow ranging from 0.5 to 5l/min o2, either approximately between 25 and 40% of the necessary oxygen supply . For a desaturation light
Mask has high concentration 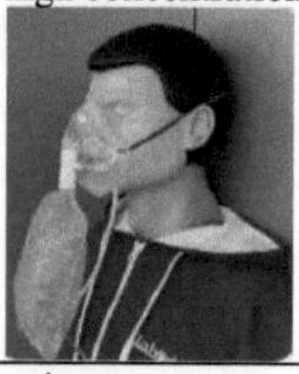	Speed : 5 – 15 L/min FiO2 = 90%For of the desaturation quite deep
Valve Boussignac 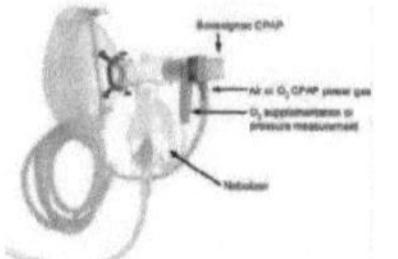	With A Speed of 15 L/min, there valve helps generate positive expiratory pressure of 5mmHg which promotes alveolar recruitment Method No invasive reserved with severe forms
Telescope nasal has high Speed 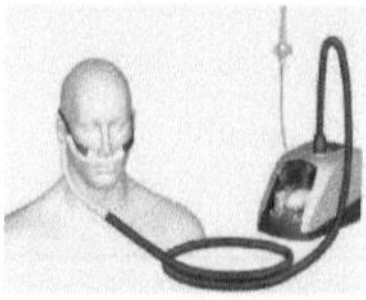	Speed Who can reach 60L/min FiO2: adjustable (up to 100%) Adjustable temperature Helps reduce dead space and promotes oxygenation of the lungs
Ventilation No invasive (NIV) 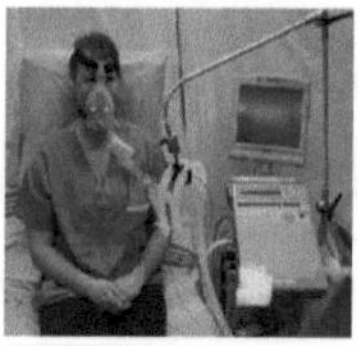	Widely used at the house of of the patients with pneumonia with pulmonary involvement > 50% Fashion Ventilation spontaneous with PEEP and adjustable pressure support Patient conscious
Ventilation mechanical (Intubation) 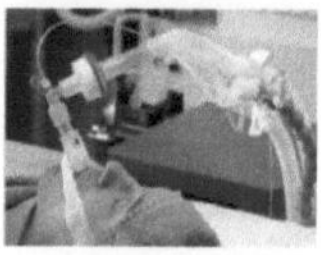	Of last appeal After failure of the others alternatives For patients in shock or sometimes For others distresses vital Ventilation of the patients in ARDS

Painting 7 : oxygen therapy in case of COVID-19 at the house of there women pregnant

7.2. THE fashion childbirth

At the start of the pandemic, and in the absence of sufficient scientific data, infection with COVID-19 alone constituted an indication for delivery by cesarean section in order to reduce maternal-fetal vertical transmission and ensure protection of healthcare personnel. health and this by analogy with the treatment protocols burden of other serious viruses such as HIV. However, it is recognized that delivery by cesarean section is associated with a high risk of incidents and accidents compared to delivery by vaginal delivery. natural such that : hemorrhage of post parturition, THE infections, THE thromboembolic diseases, the increase in the cost of care, the duration of hospitalization, without forgetting the impact psychological. The mode childbirth of a patient achievement by there COVID-19 has do of the controversies Who don't have not lasted a long time and after a few months and based on initial clinical observations, vaginal delivery was recommended as soon as possible. For these reasons, the rates of cesareans varied depending on of the pandemic period. In fact, at the start of the emergence of the virus, the rates published in the literature were between 86% and 100%. Caesarean section was the preferred method of delivery for any woman testing HIV positive (66). With the evolution of the understanding of the effects of COVID-19 infection in pregnant women, in particular the risk of vertical transmission, learned societies have agreed that cesarean section should be indicated depending on the severity of the situation. COVID and the obstetric particularities of each patient. This attitude has do fall THE rate of cesarean sections of more that 50% (67). However, these new rates remain significantly higher in comparison with the population of unaffected parturients. A systematic review including 39 studies found that between 52.3% and 95.8% of COVID patients underwent a cesarean section (96). Prabhu noted an increase in C-section birth rates even among asymptomatic COVID patients positive by report to patients No infected, with of the rate approximately 40% compared to 30% in uninfected patients (68). Metz found that an infection severe At COVID-19 was associated has A risk increased childbirth by cesarean section (59.6 % against 34.0 %, RR : 1.57, IC has 95 % : 1.30-1.90) (69). In effect the severe presentations of the infection, require rapid extraction in order to improve THE functions cardiac And respiratory of there women And to optimise thus the efficiency therapeutic in particular oxygen therapy. In series local, we have note that there cesarean section has summer practiced at the house of 64.17% of the case, And 94.11% of severe forms, which is consistent with data from the literature (46).

7.3. Impact of fashion childbirth on THE prognosis maternal

A meta-analysis led by Fatnic And al in 2023, containing 3256 case of pregnant women admitted to the delivery room and HIV positive, evaluated the effect of the mode of delivery on the evolution of the respiratory parameters of postpartum patients and gave the following results:

• In asymptomatic patients, there was a decrease in mean oxygen saturation of 1.58% in surgical patients and 0.74% in vaginally delivered patients. The use of mask oxygen therapy was more frequent in cesarean patients (4.2% versus 2.17%). None No mechanical ventilation was observed in both groups.

• In moderate forms, deterioration of the function respiratory tract was more pronounced with a decrease in average oxygen saturation of 3.98% in operated patients and 1.49% in vaginally delivered patients. The use of oxygen therapy by mask was also more frequent among patients Caesarized (12.6% versus 7.55%). Analysis multivariate, has deducted that cesarean delivery is a risk factor for respiratory deterioration in COVID-positive women (70).

Likewise, González-Castro showed in his study that ARDS was more common And more severe, at the house of THE patients given birth by cesarean sections 2.8% versus 0.78% For THE childbirth by way natural, however this study born does not specify the clinical stage of the viral pathology (71). Acute respiratory distress syndrome is an inflammatory process affecting the lungs causing nonhydrostatic, protein-rich pulmonary edema. The immediate consequences are the appearance of profound hypoxemia, a decrease in pulmonary compliance as well as an increase in intrapulmonary shunting and dead space. At the ultra-structural level, we find acute inflammation of the alveolar-capillary barrier, surfactant depletion and a reduction in pulmonary aeration.

ARDS is a criterion for the severity of pneumonia due to SARS-Cov2. His catch in charge East delicate since THE goals therapeutic initials of ARDS and septic shock may seem contradictory. Indeed, if on the hemodynamic level vascular filling, essential during cesarean section, has there phase early of shock septic East recommended, this one must be used with caution in patients with ARDS because this filling can lead to a reduction in oxygen transport and the occurrence of acute cor pulmonale (72).

Our study confirms the results of the literature: cesarean section was a factor in increased oxygen requirements (OR 6.92, 95% CI, 1.50-31.73), and acute respiratory distress syndrome (OR 4.58, CI 95 %,1.15-19.66) compared to vaginal delivery. In comparing, rates admission in resuscitation in postpartum, patients with oxygen saturation between 94 and 97% on room air, delivery by cesarean section had an increased risk of 34% compared to childbirth by way low (9%). This risk reached 46.7% when there Caesarean section is performed urgently (73). Likewise, Cavaillon showed that the use of catecholamines was more frequent In band cesarean section with GOLD : 1,562, (I.C. at 95%: 1.128-1.87) for patients with severe symptoms (74). On the other hand, there mostly of the studies don't have not watch of differences significant in the rate admission in resuscitation in function of fashion of childbirth and this regardless of the clinical picture of COVID infection (75,76).

Jarraya et al (46), reported the role of cesarean section in increasing admissions in intensive care units in postpartum (OR 5.83, 95% CI, 1.03-28.7). However This result must be interpreter with precaution, seen that This result takes not in consideration THE kind of postman of severity. In this study, COVID-positive women who had a cesarean had a greater risk of developing postpartum thrombosis (OR 2.08, 95% CI, 0.87-6.34). In the same study (46) we found that cesarean section does not constitute a postman of risk of development of a state of shock septic in post partum. Theiler carried out a single-center retrospective study including COVID women positive, No crazy, having given birth by cesarean section on a period of 4 months. This study showed that there was an increase in the incidence of a condition of shock in post parturition by report to women No crazy given birth by low track (2.81% versus 0.63%)(77). Emily H. Adhikari has accomplished a study prospective multicenter including THE women positive has there COVID-19 at the time of childbirth operated by cesarean sections " on request » And presenting with mild and moderate presentations of infection. The risk of occurrence of a State of shock septic was slightly decreases In THE band cesarean section 0.862, (I.C. has 95 % : 0,588-0,961) (78). Mahajan, evaluated the evolution of preeclampsia postpartum in COVID-positive patients at a higher term at 34 weeks, the number of patients included was of 38, none case worsening of there pathology hypertensive n / A been found. This study born precise not there classification of severity of there pathology preeclamptic (79).

Celewicz, carried out a multicenter retrospective study of cases of PE in COVID women positive wearing on 74 women, multivariate analysis showed greater risk for operated women to develop biological complications such as that there thrombocytopenia, there cytolysis hepatic And the increase of there LDH, RR :1.162, (95% CI: 0.818-1.961). This risk is not increased for clinical complications RR: 0.362, (95% CI: 0.107-0.661) (80). A Cochrane metaanalysis attempted to evaluate the impact of the mode of delivery in severe PE, excluded all studies initially collected in the COVID-positive subgroup given the heterogeneity of classifications, low numbers and selection bias. patients. This metaanalysis proposes to extrapolate data from COVID-negative women to the infected population. This analysis has concluded that childbirth by cesarean section has A effect protector from the worsening of preeclampsia, this is explained by the speed of the etiological treatment which is placental extraction, which breaks the vicious circle of the pathology.

En conclusion, la COVID-19 en elle seule ne doit jamais être une indication pour césarienne.

However, in studies including the very beginning of the pandemic where some have opted for systematic cesarean section, the absence of indication can be observed. In our multicenter observational study (46), the indications for cesarean sections were as follows:

	Effectif	Pourcentage (%)
Souffrance fœtale aigue	34	26.35%
Anomalie du travail	8	6.02%
Utérus cicatriciel	24	18.60%
Anomalie d'insertion placentaire	3	1.55%
Retard de croissance intra utérin	10	7.75%
Présentation dystocique	3	2.32%
Prééclampsie sévère	14	10.85%
Sauvetage maternel devant un tableau grave d'une infection COVID	16	12.40%
Césarienne systématique	17	13.17%

Painting 7 : Indications of cesarean section at the house of there population COVID-19 (46).

8- THERE VACCINATION AND PREGNANCY

There vaccination anti COVID-19 East a strategy safe And effective at the house of there general population (81). It has been widely recommended in pregnant and breastfeeding women (82,83) despite the non-participation of these patients in initial clinical trials (84) and has demonstrated efficacy and safety. Several learned societies have justified the vaccination at the house of the pregnant woman by the significant risk of morbidity and mortality in this population which is significantly lower with vaccination which has already shown its safety in the general population. RNA vaccines were the first to be recommended for women pregnant, until This that WHO recommended Currently a range of anti-COVID-19 vaccines. However, the pregnant woman did not participate in the therapeutic trials of the different vaccines; hence the interest in evaluating the safety and effectiveness of vaccination in pregnant women. At the start of vaccination, studies investigated the safety and security of vaccination in pregnant women even with incomplete vaccination without studying the impact on maternal and obstetric data (85). Ravit Peretz-Machluf carried out a single-center retrospective study including women Who have given birth without be affected by there COVID-19 (4700 women) (86); this study has reported safety of there vaccination on childbirth And on the fetus. However, studies which have focused on both maternal obstetric and fetal data, as is the case in our case study, are more and more frequent and further enrich the literature on the subject and present a considerable contribution to the clinical practice because they make it possible to further encourage anti-COVID vaccination in this population (87-90). It seems logical that the severity of COVID-19 will influence obstetric data And fetal seen that THE affected severe can train maternal hypoxia; severe preeclampsia which can condition the mode and indications of childbirth. Gold, all THE series of there literature are in favor of a reduction of there severity of there COVID-19 at the house of there population vaccinated This which could change the prognosis of the mother and the fetus and change the obstetric parameters in particular the mode of delivery by favoring the physiological route, hence the interest of our study on vaccination. Indeed, it has been demonstrated that immunity conferred by a primary vaccination (2 doses of vaccine to RNA) had to be restimulated At end of 6 month in reason of there decrease of antibody level necessary has there protection against infection And this has summer observed at everyone the individuals And In all slices age (91). A deadline of 6 months between primary vaccination and the booster dose (booster shot) was chosen because it has been shown that this delay is sufficient to reactivate and improve anti-COVID immunity at the population vaccinated (92). A deadline more short could be less efficient because the immune system can find itself in a state of less reactivity if it is contacted too quickly by the same antigens after the first contact. The CNOGF (National College of French Obstetricians and Gynecologists), the GRIG (Band of Research on the Infections during the Pregnancy), in France, and the ACOG (American College of Obstetricians and Gynecologists) recommend there vaccination at the house of there women pregnant And consider that one The 3rd dose of vaccine should be offered to women who are pregnant or planning to become pregnant when the initial schedule is more than 6 months old. In a prospective observational study, Jarraya et al (93), excluded women whose vaccination schedule was incomplete to avoid selection bias that could jeopardize the interpretation and validity of the results. We recall Thus that one single dose of vaccine has base RNA confers immunity of around 50% against symptomatic forms (56) linked to the Chinese strain with less effectiveness against new variants. This rate increases has more that 95% After there second dose For a duration of 6 month (5.56) In there population general THE studies have watch that there vaccination anti COVID-19 reduces the severity of the disease, the rate hospitalization, and morbidity and mortality (93).Jarraya et al (93) included only pregnant patients who required hospitalization, whether for the severity of the disease (need in oxygen distress, maternal-fetal monitoring) or peripartum hospitalization for childbirth. This will allow us to identify the differences between vaccinated and unvaccinated pregnant populations. vaccinated in terms of clinical symptoms, severity of illness, duration of hospitalization, stay in resuscitation and fetal impact. In literature he there was a lot of discussion about the impact of there COVID-19 on THE placenta And THE fetus (risk of vertical transmission, placental ischemia and alteration of maternal-fetal exchanges responsible for fetal suffering and growth retardation or even MFIU) where studies have shown the safety and benefit of vaccines. Regan NOT. Theiler has accomplished a study single-center retrospective including all women having given birth on a period of 4 month. This study showed a reduction in the incidence of disease (symptomatic COVID-19) in the vaccinated population: among the 2002 women included in this study; 140 women were vaccinated. covid 19 infection was described in two vaccinated women (2/140 :1.4%) versus 210 at the house of THE No vaccinated (210/1862 : 11.3%) (94). Others studies have watch interest of there vaccination In there reduction of the severity of covid-19. Emily H. Adhikari conducted a multicenter prospective study including all women positive for COVID-19 at the time of delivery over a two-year period. This study considers the use of oxygen therapy as a severity criterion. Among the 2641 women included in this study, 307 women had a complete vaccination schedule. 112 women developed a severe form of the disease, only 4 of whom were vaccinated (4/112 or 3.5%) (95). Joe Eid found the same results in his retrospective study including all women positive has there COVID-19 At moment of childbirth. Among THE 99 women included, 17 women were correctly vaccinated. No woman in the vaccinated group required oxygen therapy, however. 22% of women no vaccinated have need of O2 (96). Haemin Kim has accomplished a study retrospective comparing a group of vaccinated pregnant women (39 women) versus A band of women speakers no vaccinated (185 women). THE vaccinated women were mostly asymptomatic Or affected of a shape minor in 94.9% of cases. Vaccination has made it possible to reduce the use of oxygen therapy in the group of vaccinated women from 16.2% to 2.6% (97). Samantha NOT. Piekos has accomplished a study retrospective multicenter including all women who gave birth in the centers participating in the study (86,833 women including 48,492 unvaccinated). COVID -19 infection was diagnosed in 916 women vaccinated versus 3394 unvaccinated women (p<0.001). So, THE rate infection has there COVID-19 at the house of THE vaccinated has been reduced. However, this study did not find a difference in the use of hospitalization but showed a reduced need for oxygen therapy (98). Currently, he There are meta-analyses that showed an association between COVID-19 and the occurrence of preeclampsia (99,100) it East known that the infection to the COVID-19 in women pregnant increase her rate ,this has been explained by placental ischemia and decidual arteriopathy with thromboses (101,102). Shu Qin Wei's meta-analysis of 42 studies including 438,548 women pregnant do The example, he has find that comparatively has the absence of infection by THE SARS-CoV-2 during there pregnancy, THE diagnostic of COVID-19 has summer partner has there preeclampsia (OR= 1.33; IC has 95 % 1.03–1.73) And that by compared to minor forms of COVID-19, the Severe COVID-19 was more strongly associated with preeclampsia (OR = 4.16; 95% CI 1.55–11.15) (103).Vaccination did not increase the rate of preeclampsia relative to the population No COVID-19, this has summer widely proven In of the studies to wide scales (104,105). Regan N. Theiler (94) previously found that vaccination was associated with a nonsignificant decrease in the incidence of preeclampsia (0.7% versus 1.2% RR: 0.58; 95% CI, 0.08–4.25; p = 0.59). Jarray et al reported a difference between the two groups in terms of preeclampsia (93). Our results are comparable with those of there literature which still remains controversial on the reduction in the incidence of preeclampsia associated with COVID-19 during pregnancy in the vaccinated population. As for cytolysis associated with

COVID-19, we noted a decrease of the incidence of the hepatic cytolysis in the group " vaccinated " of 16% has 6.6% without this drop being significant. In effect he Cytolysis has been shown to be an indicator of severity and poor maternal prognosis (106). Several studies have looked for the impact of COVID-19 on the rate of cesarean sections (107) At the start of the pandemic, it appears that the rate of cesarean sections was higher (108). This could be explained by the absence of clinical data on the impact of mode of delivery on fetal and maternal prognosis. In this period COVID-19 alone was reported as an indication for cesarean section under several pretexts such that there reduction of risk of transmission vertical (109). Afterwards, At course of there pandemic, And After to have known THE risk increased of morbidity linked to cesarean section, learned societies formally recommend respecting the obstetric and fetal indications for cesarean section. In addition, the advent of vaccination has certainly reduces the severity of painting clinical of the COVID-19 can change the prognosis of patients and subsequently influence the mode of delivery (46). Several studies have reported an increase in the rate of cesarean sections for fetal distress in unvaccinated parturients (110,111) while others have not found an impact of vaccination on the mode of delivery. (112). This stay always one subject of controversies especially since there are selection biases in quite a few studies, especially those which included patients with incomplete vaccination. There are numerous studies that have looked at the impact of vaccination on maternal complications (52,58). The majority of these studies did not find a reduction in the incidence of postpartum complications. This could be explained by postoperative rehabilitation protocols which have shown their effectiveness in reducing postoperative complications (113).

In addition, the series in the literature, especially those from the start of vaccination, are of limited size and are most often retrospective studies which report the experience of the different teams and country without as much specify the method for calculating the sample size and without specifying the statistical power of these studies And their validity For detect THE differences in terms of morbidity linked to childbirth. It has been reported that maternal and fetal prognosis essentially depends of there severity of the storm cytokine (114), Who could be less significant in vaccinated women. This was a strong argument for thinking about a reduction of there maternal morbidity in postpartum at the house of the vaccinated. In our study, there vaccination has reduced THE rate of the cesarean sections in decreasing there severity of illness; and the rate of acute fetal suffering, which has allowed more vaginal deliveries outside of urgent indications for cesarean sections, this can reduce the incidence of the risks related to anesthesia (115), postpartum hemorrhage and thromboembolic events and may improve recovery after delivery (116,117). In our study, vaccination made it possible to reduce the duration of hospitalization of affected parturients. by there COVID-19. In effect, he exist little of studies Who have studied the impact of vaccination on this parameter. This could be explained by the subjectivity of this parameter to judge the impact of vaccination because it depends closely on the conducts of the patricians Who different certainly of a team has the other but also At breast from the same team. However, Studies carried out in the general population have reported a reduction in the length of hospitalization, intensive care unit stay and morbidity and mortality in the vaccinated population (118,119). At the house of THE women pregnant, several studies (120,121) have watch that the vaccination reduced THE risks of mortality by there COVID-19 despite his vulnerability has this virus (122) And there presence of a risk increased of stay in intensive care and mortality (123). Hence the great contribution and clinical interest of vaccination Who has become more and more more recommended in this population. In a study multicenter doing participate 6 country (United Kingdom, Netherlands, Norway, Denmark, Finland And Italy) on there period between May And December 2021, it was shown that the stay in intensive care was significantly reduced by vaccination as well as maternal mortality from COVID-19

(120,121). In OUR study (93), there vaccination has permit of decrease there mortality kindergarten without that this decrease born either significant. We let's think that there size of the sample of OUR series born allow not of clear of the differences significant on A event (there mortality kindergarten) of which there frequency was lower has 2% at THE women No vaccinated according to THE different series of there literature (120,121). In more, THE case unique of mortality kindergarten at the house of there The vaccinated population of this series had a heavy comorbidity with a very severe form of preeclampsia (HELLP syndrome). Remember that maternal mortality is still a public health problem in developing countries even outside of COVID-19.

9- THERE VACCINATION HAS THE ERA OF THERE VARIANT " OMICRON » OF SARS COV2

Indeed, within the Omicron variant, multiple mutations of the Spike protein, characteristic of SARS-CoV-2 and main target of vaccines (124), suggest to a lower effectiveness of vaccination initially designed to attack there strain savage of virus appeared in China in 2019. He is of a virus that risks evading COVID-19 vaccines and treatments. Several studies (124,125) have demonstrated the reduced effectiveness of neutralizing antibodies on this variant. In addition, the low virulence of the Omicron variant, responsible for an attenuation of symptoms even in the absence of vaccination in pregnant women (93), has led to the trivialization of the disease. and a forgetting of vaccination, hence the interest in clinical studies evaluating the effectiveness of there vaccination anti-COVID-19 has the era of there variant Omicron (126). Faced with successive mutations of the virus each time generating a different strain (21), nature will select the virus that is most contagious for humans. independently of there severity of there disease that he go generate. In more, and in front identification of co-infections (127) by of the strains different at the house of the same individual, the risk of obtaining a recombinant virus with different genomes exists. This could achieve has a new strain recombinant there contagiousness of Omicron and the clinical severity of Delta (128,129). In more, THE good results of there vaccination And there decrease natural of there severity of there disease with THE news variants, has pushed there population to give less importance has there vaccination. A relaxation Who begin has to touch even practitioners and hospital structures, especially since certain authors and experts believe that the Omicron variant heralds the end of the pandemic (130). But unfortunately the end of tunnel is not not Again there. We wish warn the authors of the probable risks of this enigma infection which never ceases to surprise us And THE encourage has TO DO of the studies on efficiency of vaccine against the news variants Who exist Currently. He seems that recommend a booster dose of the vaccine (booster dose) during pregnancy seems reasonable, especially after the latest encouraging clinical results for the mother and the newborn (128-130). He seems Also careful of born not to leave to fall THE measurements of protection individual And having of the circuits And of the units isolation COVID-19 obstetrics ready has employment has anything what moment (131). We we also mention the interest of a continuous evaluation of the role of vaccination on the disease in the mother as well as in the fetus and the newborn given the changing aspect of COVID-19 and the emergence of new strains to each wave (129,130).

In a study recent, Jarraya And al have watch that THE women having had a 3rd dose of vaccine during of there pregnancy had of best results by report to those who have had only 2 doses (131), hence the interest in giving vaccine boosters every 6 months and preferably a booster dose At 3rd [trimester] in order to obtain of the antibody Who are going by there following pass towards THE fetus And ensure more safety for the newborn. Regarding fetal data, studies by Jarraya et al (93,126) showed an increased incidence of admissions to neonatal intensive care settings of newborns born to unvaccinated mothers. Several studies have demonstrated that vaccination during pregnancy a double benefit. It provides protection for the mother as well only for her newborn who can cover the 6 first months of life (133,134). THE children of down ages Who born are not eligible for COVID-19 vaccination so far, represent a population at risk of developing severe forms of SARS-CoV-2 as well as formidable complications, not yet well understood, of this disease, of which we cite multi-systemic inflammatory syndrome (MIS-C) (135).An American multicenter study carried out in 30 hospitals in 22 American states published in June 2022, correlated vaccine effectiveness during pregnancy At risk hospitalization of the children For COVID-19 And This during the circulation of the variants Delta And Omicron. They have defined a vaccination complete in pregnant parturients by the administration of 2 doses of mRNA vaccine (BNT162b2 [Pfizer–BioNTech]

And mRNA-1273 [Moderna]). They have demonstrated that vaccination during pregnancy reduces the risk of hospitalization of children, whose age is less than 6 months, by 80% during the Delta wave and by 38% during the Omicron wave. Vaccine effectiveness against transfer to intensive care settings in children was 70%. In addition, 90% of children admitted to intensive care units were from unvaccinated mothers (134). These results are consistent with the results of our study (126). This study and other studies (136) were able to show that the antibodies obtained through vaccination are transferable to newborns and are indeed effective in conferring protection covering At less THE 6 first month of life. There vaccination kindergarten by 2 doses of vaccines has mRNA during there Omicron wave stay associated to a reduction judged moderate of risk hospitalization at the house of THE infants, and this, explained by the low neutralization of antibodies against this variant further emphasizing the importance of administering booster doses in pregnant women as in the general population (134). On the other hand, protection humoral passively transferable to newborns via THE milk maternal has summer confirmed by a cohort German Who analyzed THE rate antibodies in the serum And In THE milk maternal of the parturients having summer previously infected with the virus or vaccinated during pregnancy. This team concluded to the presence of antibodies anti-COVID 19 In THE milk maternal of which efficiency of neutralization concerns even there variant Omicron And adds that THE title THE more pupil of antibodies was observed at the house of the women convalescents of the infection during there pregnancy and who received a dose of vaccine while breastfeeding (137). For this reason, breastfeeding should always be encouraged as it could improve the newborn's immunity and reduce the risks related to COVID -19.

REFERENCES

1. de Medeiros KS, Sarmento ACA, Costa APF, al. Consequences and implications of the coronavirus disease (COVID-19) on pregnancy and newborns: A comprehensive systematic review and meta-analysis. Int J Gynaecol Obstet. March 2022;156(3):394-405.

2. Liu Y, Chen H, Tan W, et al. Clinical characteristics and outcome of SARS-CoV-2 infection during pregnancy. J Infect. June 2021;82(6):e9-10.

3. Areia AL, Mota-Pinto A. Can immunity during pregnancy influence SARS-CoV-2 infection? - A systematic review. J Reprod Immunol. Nov 2020;142:103215.

4. Jamieson DJ, Rasmussen SA. An update on COVID-19 and pregnancy. Am J Obstet Gynecol. févr 2022;226(2):177-86.

5. Castro P, Matos AP, Werner H, et al. Covid-19 and Pregnancy: An Overview. Rev Bras Ginecol Obstet. juill 2020;42(7):420-6.

6. Birol Ilter P, Prasad S, Berkkan M, et al. Clinical severity of SARS-CoV-2 infection among vaccinated and unvaccinated pregnancies during the Omicron wave. Ultrasound Obstet Gynecol. avr 2022;59(4):560-2.

7. Di Martino D, Chiaffarino F, Patanè L, et al. Assessing risk factors for severe forms of COVID-19 in a pregnant population: A clinical series from Lombardy, Italy. Int J Gynaecol Obstet. févr 2021;152(2):275-7.

8. Miyamoto M, Perreand E, Mangione M, et al. Mode of Delivery in Patients with COVID- 19. Am J Obstet Gynecol. Janv 2022;226(1):S582-3.

9. Wastnedge EAN, Reynolds RM, van Boeckel SR, et al. Pregnancy and COVID-19. Physiol Rev. 1 janv 2021;101(1):303-18.

10. Thompson JL, Nguyen LM, Noble KN, et al. COVID-19-related disease severity in pregnancy. Am J Reprod Immunol. nov 2020;84(5):e13339.

11. Di Guardo F, Di Grazia FM, Di Gregorio LM, et al. Poor maternal-neonatal outcomes in pregnant patients with confirmed SARS-Cov-2 infection:

analysis of 145 cases. Arch Gynecol Obstet. juin 2021;303(6):1483-8.

12. Hantoushzadeh S, Nabavian SM, Soleimani Z, et al. COVID-19 Disease During Pregnancy and Peripartum Period: A Cardiovascular Review. Curr Probl Cardiol. Janv 2022;47(1):100888.

13. Shi Y, Wang Y, Shao C, et al. COVID-19 infection: the perspectives on immune responses. Cell Death Differ. mai 2020;27(5):1451-4.

14. Nile SH, Nile A, Qiu J, et al. COVID-19: Pathogenesis, cytokine storm and therapeutic potential of interferons. Cytokine Growth Factor Rev. juin 2020;53:66-70.

15. Rad HS, Röhl J, Stylianou N, et al. The Effects of COVID-19 on the Placenta During Pregnancy. Front Immunol. 2021 Sep 15;12:743022. doi: 10.3389/fimmu.2021.743022.

16. Bonny V, Maillard A, Mousseaux C, et al. COVID-19: physiopathology of a disease with many faces. The Journal of Internal Medicine. 2020 Jun 1;41(6):375-89.

17. Leentjens J, van Haaps TF, Wessels PF, et al. COVID-19- associated coagulopathy and antithrombotic agents—lessons after 1 year. Lancet Haematol. Jul 2021;8(7):e524-33.

18. Volpe N, Luca Schera GB, Dall'Asta A, et al. COVID-19 in pregnancy: where are we now? J Perinat Med. Jul 27, 2021;49(6):637-42.

18. Dong L, Tian J, He S, et al. Possible Vertical Transmission of SARS-CoV-2 From an Infected Mother to Her Newborn. JAMA. 12 mai 2020;323(18):1846-8.

19. Zeng H, Xu C, Fan J, et al. Antibodies in Infants Born to Mothers With COVID-19 Pneumonia. JAMA. 12 mai 2020;323(18):1848-9.

20. Bergmann CC, Silverman RH. COVID-19: Coronavirus replication, pathogenesis, and therapeutic strategies. Cleve Clin J Med. 2020 Jun;87(6):321-327

21. JarrayaA, KammounM, Bouhamed O, et al. Maternal and perinatal outcomes in the COVID-19 Omicron wave in comparison with the Delta wave: a multicentre observational study. Ital J Gynaecol Obstet 2023; 35 (3): 397-405. doi: 10.36129/jog.2022.74

22. **Kammoun, M., Jarraya, A., Hammemi, F et al.** COVID-19 Severity Among Non- Vaccinated Pregnant Women During the Delta Wave in Tunisia: A Retrospective Monocentric Study. Journal of Internal Medicine Research & Reports. SRC/JIMRR-118. DOI: doi. org/10.47363/JIMRR/2022 (1), 118.

23. **Jarraya A, Kammoun M, Dammak S, et al.** Management of COVID-19-Associated Guillain-Barré Syndrome in a Full-Term Pregnant Woman: A Case Report. Journal of Mother and Child. 2023 Jun 1;27(1):52-4.

24. **Lassi ZS, Ana A, Das JK, et al.** A systematic review and meta-analysis of data on pregnant women with confirmed COVID-19: Clinical presentation, and pregnancy and perinatal outcomes based on COVID-19 severity. J Glob Health. 30 juin 2021;11:05018.

25. **Bastos SNMAN, Barbosa BLF, Cruz LGB, et al.** Clinical and Obstetric Aspects of Pregnant Women with COVID-19: A Systematic Review. Rev Bras Ginecol Obstet. déc 2021;43(12):949-60.

26. **Chi J, Gong W, Gao Q.** Clinical characteristics and outcomes of pregnant women with COVID-19 and the risk of vertical transmission: a systematic review. Arch Gynecol Obstet. 2021;303(2):337-345.

27. **Elshafeey F, Magdi R, Hindi N, et al.** A systematic scoping review of COVID-19 during pregnancy and childbirth. Int J Gynaecol Obstet. Juill 2020;150(1):47-52.

28. **Vouga M, Favre G, Martinez-Perez O, et al.** Maternal outcomes and risk factors for COVID-19 severity among pregnant women. Sci Rep. 6 juill 2021;11:13898.

29. **Allotey J, Fernandez S, Bonet M, et al.** Clinical manifestations, risk factors, and maternal and perinatal outcomes of coronavirus disease 2019 in pregnancy: living systematic review and meta-analysis. BMJ. 1 sept 2020;370:m3320.

30. Tutiya C, Mello F, Chaccur G, et al. Risk factors for severe and critical Covid-19 in pregnant women in a single center in Brazil. The Journal of Maternal-Fetal & Neonatal Medicine. 12 déc 2022;35(25):5389-92.

31. Menezes MO, Takemoto MLS, Nakamura-Pereira M, et al. Risk factors for adverse outcomes among pregnant and postpartum women with acute respiratory distress syndrome due to COVID-19 in Brazil. Int J Gynaecol Obstet. déc 2020;151(3):415-23.

32. Ko JY, DeSisto CL, Simeone RM, et al. Adverse Pregnancy Outcomes, Maternal Complications, and Severe Illness Among US Delivery Hospitalizations With and Without a Coronavirus Disease 2019 (COVID-19) Diagnosis. Clin Infect Dis. 15 juill 2021;73(Suppl 1):S24-31.

33. Pierce-Williams RAM, Burd J, Felder L, et al. Clinical course of severe and critical coronavirus disease 2019 in hospitalized pregnancies: a United States cohort study. Am J Obstet Gynecol MFM. août 2020;2(3):100134.

34. Wu Y, Li H, Guo X, et al. Incidence, risk factors, and prognosis of abnormal liver biochemical tests in COVID-19 patients: a systematic review and meta-analysis. Hepatol Int. 24 juill 2020;14(5):621-37.

35. Molteni E, Astley CM, Ma W, et al. Symptoms and syndromes associated with SARS- CoV-2 infection and severity in pregnant women from two community cohorts. Sci Rep. 25 mars 2021;11(1):6928.

36. Zhu X, Song B, Shi F, et al. Joint prediction and time estimation of COVID-19 developing severe symptoms using chest CT scan. Med Image Anal. Janv 2021;67:101824.

37.Zhang K, Liu X, Shen J, et al. Clinically Applicable AI System for Accurate Diagnosis, Quantitative Measurements, and Prognosis of COVID-19 Pneumonia Using Computed Tomography. Cell. 11 juin 2020;181(6):1423-1433.e11.

38. Wei SQ, Bilodeau-Bertrand M, Liu S, et al . The impact of COVID-19 on pregnancy outcomes: a systematic review and meta-analysis. CMAJ Can Med

Assoc J J Assoc Medicale Can. 19 avr 2021;193(16):E540-8.

39 . Soldavini CM, Di Martino D, Sabattini E, et al. sFlt-1/PlGF ratio in hypertensive disorders of pregnancy in patients affected by COVID-19. Pregnancy Hypertens. 2022;27:103-9.

40. Shanes ED, Mithal LB, Otero S, et al. Placental Pathology in COVID-19. Am J Clin Pathol. juin 2020;154(1):23-32.

41. Regitz-Zagrosek V, Roos-Hesselink JW, Bauersachs J, et al. 2018 ESC Guidelines for the management of cardiovascular diseases during pregnancy. Eur Heart J. 7 sept 2018;39(34):3165-241.

42. Baracy M, Afzal F, Szpunar SM, et al. Coronavirus disease 2019 (COVID-19) and the risk of hypertensive disorders of pregnancy: a retrospective cohort study. Hypertens Pregnancy. Août 2021;40(3):226-35.

43. Madden N, Emeruwa UN, Polin M, et al. SARS-CoV-2 and hypertensive disease in pregnancy. Am J Obstet Gynecol Mfm. janv 2022;4(1):100496.

44. Jering KS, Claggett BL, Cunningham JW, et al. Clinical Characteristics and Outcomes of Hospitalized Women Giving Birth With and Without COVID-19. JAMA Intern Med. Mai 2021;181(5):714-7.

45. Conde-Agudelo A, Romero R. SARS-CoV-2 infection during pregnancy and risk of preeclampsia: a systematic review and meta-analysis. Am J Obstet Gynecol. janv 2022;226(1):68-89.e3.

46. Jarraya A, Kammoun M, Bouhamed O, et al. The impact of the mode of delivery on the prognosis of pregnant women with COVID-19: a multicentre observational study. . Ital J Gynaecol Obstet 2023; 35 (3): 367-374 doi: 10.36129/jog.2022.72

47. Martin JA, Hamilton BE, Osterman MJ. Births in the United States, 2021. NCHS Data Brief. août 2022;(442):1-8.

48. Ellington S, Strid P, Tong VT, et al. Characteristics of Women of Reproductive Age with Laboratory- Confirmed SARS-CoV-2 Infection by Pregnancy Status — United States, January 22–June 7, 2020. Morb Mortal Wkly

Rep. 26 juin 2020;69(25):769-75.

49. Zambrano LD, Ellington S, Strid P, et al. Update: Characteristics of Symptomatic Women of Reproductive Age with Laboratory-Confirmed SARS-CoV-2 Infection by Pregnancy Status
— United States, January 22–October 3, 2020. Morb Mortal Wkly Rep. 6 nov 2020;69(44):1641-7.

50. Madjunkov M, Dviri M, Librach C. A comprehensive review of the impact of COVID- 19 on human reproductive biology, assisted reproduction care and pregnancy: a Canadian perspective. J Ovarian Res. 27 nov 2020;13(1):140.

51. Leung C, Su L, Simões E Silva AC. Better healthcare can reduce the risk of COVID-19 in-hospital post-partum maternal death: evidence from Brazil. Int J Epidemiol. 13 déc 2022;51(6):1733-44.

52. Rahayuwati L, Nurhidayah I, Ekawati R, et al. Determinant Factors of Post-Partum Contraception among Women during COVID-19 in West Java Province, Indonesia. Int J Environ Res Public Health. 28 janv 2023;20(3):2303.

53. Dashraath P, Nielsen-Saines K, Rimoin A, et al. Monkeypox in pregnancy: virology, clinical presentation, and obstetric management. Am J Obstet Gynecol. déc 2022;227(6):849- 861.e7.

53. Kahankova R, Barnova K, Jaros R, et al. Pregnancy in the time of COVID-19: towards Fetal monitoring 4.0. BMC Pregnancy Childbirth. 16 janv 2023;23(1):33.

54. Zayyan S, Frise C. COVID-19 in pregnancy: A UK perspective. Obstet Med. déc 2022;15(4):216-9.

55. Ramos A, Joaquin C, Ros M, et al. Impact of COVID-19 on nutritional status during the first wave of the pandemic. Clin Nutr Edinb Scotl. déc 2022;41(12):3032-7.

56. Yan J, Guo J, Fan C, et al. Coronavirus disease 2019 in pregnant women: a report based on 116 cases. Am J Obstet Gynecol. Juill 2020;223(1):111.e1-

111.e14.

57. Gurol-Urganci I, Jardine JE, Carroll F, et al. Maternal and perinatal outcomes of pregnant women with SARS-CoV-2 infection at the time of birth in England: national cohort study. Am J Obstet Gynecol. nov 2021;225(5):522.e1-522.e11.

58. Ahlberg M, Neovius M, Saltvedt S, et al. Association of SARS-CoV-2 Test Status and Pregnancy Outcomes.
JAMA. 3 nov 2020;324(17):1782-5.

59. Delahoy MJ, Whitaker M, O'Halloran A, et al. Characteristics and Maternal and Birth Outcomes of Hospitalized Pregnant Women with Laboratory-Confirmed COVID-19 — COVID-NET, 13 States, March 1–August 22, 2020. Morb Mortal Wkly Rep. 25 sept 2020;69(38):1347-54.

60. Vergara-Merino L, Meza N, et al. Maternal and perinatal outcomes related to COVID-19 and pregnancy: An overview of systematic reviews. Acta Obstet Gynecol Scand. juill 2021;100(7):1200-18.

61. Vousden N, Bunch K, Morris E, et al. The incidence, characteristics and outcomes of pregnant women hospitalized with symptomatic and asymptomatic SARS-CoV-2 infection in the UK from March to September 2020: A national cohort study using the UK Obstetric Surveillance System (UKOSS). PLoS ONE. 5 mai 2021;16(5):e0251123.

62. Lye P, Dunk CE, Zhang J, et al. ACE2 Is Expressed in Immune Cells That Infiltrate the Placenta in Infection-Associated Preterm Birth. Cells. 8 juill 2021;10(7):1724.

63. Al-Kuraishy HM, Al-Gareeb AI, Albezrah NKA, et al. Pregnancy and COVID-19: high or low risk of vertical transmission. Clin Exp Med. 17 oct 2022;1-11.

64. Garcia-Flores V, Romero R, Xu Y, et al. Maternal-Fetal Immune Responses in Pregnant Women Infected with SARS-CoV-2. Res Sq. 31 mars 2021;rs.3.rs-362886.

65. **Öcal DF, Öztürk FH, Şenel SA, et al.** The influence of COVID-19 pandemic on intrauterine fetal demise and possible vertical transmission of SARS-CoV-2. Taiwan J Obstet Gynecol. Nov 2022;61(6):1021-6.

66- **Simsek Y, Ciplak B, Songur S, et al.** Maternal and fetal outcomes of COVID-19, SARS, and MERS: a narrative review on the current knowledge. Eur Rev Med Pharmacol Sci. sept 2020;24(18):9748-52.

67- **Giuliani F, Deantoni S, Papageorghiou AT**. Vaginal vs cesarean delivery for COVID-19 in pregnancy. Am J Obstet Gynecol. mars 2023;228(3):358-9.

68- **Prabhu M, Cagino K, Matthews KC, et al.** Pregnancy and postpartum outcomes in a universally tested population for SARS-CoV-2 in New York City: a prospective cohort study. BJOG Int J Obstet Gynaecol. nov 2020;127(12):1548-56.

69- **Metz TD, Clifton RG, Hughes BL, et al.** Disease Severity and Perinatal Outcomes of Pregnant Patients With Coronavirus Disease 2019 (COVID-19). Obstet Gynecol. Avr 2021;137(4):571-80.

70. **Fatnic E, Blanco NL, Cobiletchi R, et al**. Outcome predictors and patient progress following delivery in pregnant and postpartum patients with severe COVID-19 pneumonitis in intensive care units in Israel (OB-COVICU): a nationwide cohort study. Lancet Respir Med. Juin 2023;11(6):520-9.

71. **González-Castro A, Martos Benítez FD, Fernández-Rodríguez A, et al.** [Validation of the P/FPe index in to cohort of patients with ARDS secondary to SARS-CoV-2]. Med Intensive. Juill 2023;47(7):413-5.

72. **Zhang J, Pang Q, Zhou T, et al**. Risk factors for acute kidney injury in COVID-19 patients: an updated systematic review and meta-analysis. Ren Fail. déc 2023;45(1):2170809.

73. **Bellanti F, Kasperczyk S, Kasperczyk A, et al.** Alteration of circulating redox balance in coronavirus disease- 19-induced acute respiratory distress syndrome. J Intensive Care. 5 juill 2023;11(1):30.

74.**Cavaillon JM.** During Sepsis and COVID-19, the Pro-Inflammatory and

Anti- Inflammatory Responses Are Concomitant. Clin Rev Allergy Immunol. 3 juill 2023;

75. van Dam M, van Hamersvelt H, Schoonhoven L, et al. Clinical supervision under pressure: a qualitative study amongst health care professionals working on the ICU during COVID-19. Med Educ Online. déc 2023;28(1):2231614.

76. Serafini A, Palandri L, Kurotschka PK, et al. The effects of primary care monitoring strategies on COVID-19 related hospitalisation and mortality: a retrospective electronic medical records review in a northern Italian province, the MAGMA study. Eur J Gen Pract. Déc 2023;29(2):2186395.

77. Theiler RN, Wick M, Mehta R, et al. Pregnancy and birth outcomes after SARS-CoV-2 vaccination in pregnancy. Am J Obstet Gynecol MFM. nov 2021;3(6):100467.

78. Adhikari EH, Spong CY. Understanding Acute Obstetric Morbidity Associated With SARS-CoV-2 Variants-Unwrapping the Layers of an Onion. JAMA Netw Open. 1 août 2022;5(8):e2226444.

79. Mahajan NN, Kesarwani S, Kumbhar P, et al. Increased risk of early-onset preeclampsia in pregnant women with COVID-19. Hypertens Pregnancy. déc 2023;42(1):2187630.

80. Celewicz A, Celewicz M, Michalczyk M, et al. SARS CoV-2 infection as a risk factor of preeclampsia and pre-term birth. An interplay between viral infection, pregnancy-specific immune shift and endothelial dysfunction may lead to negative pregnancy outcomes. Ann Med. déc 2023;55(1):2197289.

81. Ma Y, Deng J, Liu Q, et al. Effectiveness and Safety of COVID-19 Vaccine among Pregnant Women in Real-World Studies: A Systematic Review and Meta-Analysis. Vaccines. 6 févr 2022;10(2):246.

82. Galanis P, Vraka I, Siskou O, et al. Uptake of COVID-19 Vaccines among Pregnant Women: A Systematic Review and Meta-Analysis. Vaccines. 12 mai 2022;10(5):766.

83. **Taylor MM, Kobeissi L, Kim C, et al.** Inclusion of pregnant women in COVID-19 treatment trials: a review and global call to action. Lancet Glob Health. mars 2021;9(3):e366-71.

84. **Jamieson DJ, Rasmussen SA**. An update on COVID-19 and pregnancy. Am J Obstet Gynecol. 1 févr 2022;226(2):177-86.

85. **Sadarangani M, Soe P, Shulha HP, et al.** Safety of COVID-19 vaccines in pregnancy: a Canadian National Vaccine Safety (CANVAS) network cohort study. Lancet Infect Dis. 11 août 2022;S1473-3099(22)00426-1.

86. **Peretz-Machluf R, Hirsh-Yechezkel G, Zaslavsky-Paltiel I, et al.** Obstetric and Neonatal Outcomes following COVID-19 Vaccination in Pregnancy. J Clin Med. 30 avr 2022;11(9):2540.

87. **Morgan JA, Biggio JR, Martin JK, et al.** Maternal Outcomes After Severe Acute Respiratory Syndrome Coronavirus 2 (SARS-CoV-2) Infection in Vaccinated Compared With Unvaccinated Pregnant Patients. Obstet Gynecol. 1 janv 2022;139(1):107-9.

88. **Birol Ilter P, Prasad S, Berkkan M, et al.** Clinical severity of SARS-CoV-2 infection among vaccinated and unvaccinated pregnancies during the Omicron wave. Ultrasound Obstet Gynecol. avr 2022;59(4):560-2.

89. **Wang PH, Lee WL, Yang ST, et al.** The impact of COVID-19 in pregnancy: Part II. Vaccination to pregnant women. J Chin Med Assoc JCMA. 1 oct 2021;84(10):903-10.

90. **Prasad S, Kalafat E, Blakeway H, et al.** Systematic review and meta-analysis of the effectiveness and perinatal outcomes of COVID-19 vaccination in pregnancy. Nat Commun. 10 mai 2022;13(1):2414.

91. **Béné MC, Bittencourt M de C, Chevallier P.** Post-SARS-CoV-2 vaccination

specific antibody decrease : Let's get the half-full glass perspective. J Infect. 1 janv 2022;84(1):94-118.

92. **Suthar MS, Arunachalam PS, Hu M, et al.** Durability of immune

responses to the BNT162b2 mRNA vaccine. Med. 14 janv 2022;3(1):25-7.

93. Jarraya A, Kammoun M, Amouri S, et al. Impact of COVID-19 vaccination among pregnant women requiring hospital admission: prospective observational research. . Ital J Gynaecol Obstet. 2023; 35 (2) : 211-218. doi: 10.36129/jog.2022.53

94. Theiler RN, Wick M, Mehta R, et al. Pregnancy and birth outcomes after SARS-CoV-2 vaccination in pregnancy. Am J Obstet Gynecol Mfm. nov 2021;3(6):100467.

95. Adhikari EH, MacDonald L, SoRelle JA, et al. COVID-19 Cases and Disease Severity in Pregnancy and Neonatal Positivity Associated With Delta (B.1.617.2) and Omicron (B.1.1.529) Variant Predominance. JAMA. 19 avr 2022;327(15):1500-2.

96. Eid J, Abdelwahab M, Caplan M, et al. Increasing oxygen requirements and disease severity in pregnant individuals with the SARS-CoV-2 Delta variant. Am J Obstet Gynecol Mfm. mai 2022;4(3):100612.

97. Kim H, Kim HS, Kim HM, et al. Impact of vaccination and the omicron variant on COVID-19 severity in pregnant women. Am J Infect Control. 31 juill 2022;S0196- 6553(22)00592-2.

98. Piekos SN, Hwang YM, Roper RT, et al. The effect of COVID-19 vaccination and booster on maternal-fetal outcomes: a retrospective multicenter cohort study. MedRxiv Prepr Serv Health Sci. 18 août 2022;2022.08.12.22278727.

99. Conde-Agudelo A, Romero R. SARS-CoV-2 infection during pregnancy and risk of preeclampsia: a systematic review and meta-analysis. Am J Obstet Gynecol. janv 2022;226(1):68-89.e3.

100. Aho Glele LS, Simon E, Bouit C, et al. Association between SARS-Cov-2 infection during pregnancy and adverse pregnancy outcomes: A re-analysis of the data reported by Wei et al. (2021). Infect Dis Now. mai 2022;52(3):123-8.

101. Papageorghiou AT, Deruelle P, Gunier RB, et al. Preeclampsia and

COVID-19: results from the INTERCOVID prospective longitudinal study. Am J Obstet Gynecol. sept 2021;225(3):289.e1-289.e17.

102. Villar J, Ariff S, Gunier RB, et al. Maternal and Neonatal Morbidity and Mortality Among Pregnant Women With and Without COVID-19 Infection: The INTERCOVID Multinational Cohort Study. JAMA Pediatr. 1 août 2021;175(8):817-26.

103. Wei SQ, Bilodeau-Bertrand M, Liu S, Auger N. Impact of COVID-19 on pregnancy outcomes: systematic review and meta-analysis. CMAJ Can Med Assoc J. May 31, 2021;193(22):E813-22.

104. Blakeway H, Prasad S, Kalafat E, et al. COVID-19 vaccination during pregnancy: coverage and safety. Am J Obstet Gynecol. Feb 2022;226(2):236.e1-236.e14.

105. Bookstein Peretz S, Regev N, Novick L, and al. Short-term outcome of pregnant women vaccinated with BNT162b2 mRNA COVID-19 vaccine. Ultrasound Obstet Gynecol Off J Int Soc Ultrasound Obstet Gynecol. Sep 2021;58(3):450-6.

106. Yip TCF, Lui GCY, Wong VWS, et al. Liver injury is independently associated with adverse clinical outcomes in patients with COVID-19. Gut. 1 avr 2021;70(4):733-42.

107. Wei SQ, Bilodeau-Bertrand M, Liu S, et al. The impact of COVID-19 on pregnancy outcomes: a systematic review and meta-analysis. CMAJ Can Med Assoc J. 19 avr 2021;193(16):E540-8.

108. Debrabandere ML, Farabaugh DC, Giordano C. A Review on Mode of Delivery during COVID-19 between December 2019 and April 2020. Am J Perinatol. 2021;332-41.

109. Smith V, Seo D, Warty R, et al. Maternal and neonatal outcomes associated with COVID- 19 infection: A systematic review. PloS One. 2020;15(6):e0234187.

110. **Zaigham M, Andersson O.** Maternal and perinatal outcomes with

COVID-19: A systematic review of 108 pregnancies. Acta Obstet Gynecol Scand. Juill 2020;99(7):823-9.

111. Chen L, Li Q, Zheng D, et al. Clinical Characteristics of Pregnant Women with Covid- 19 in Wuhan, China. N Engl J Med. 18 juin 2020;382(25):e100.

112. Cai J, Tang M, Gao Y, et al. Cesarean Section or Vaginal Delivery to Prevent Possible Vertical Transmission From a Pregnant Mother Confirmed With COVID-19 to a Neonate: A Systematic Review. Front Med. 17 févr 2021;8:634949.

113. Eleje GU, Ugwu EO, Enebe JT, et al. Cesarean section rate and outcomes during and before the first wave of COVID-19 pandemic. SAGE Open Med. 23 mars 2022;10:20503121221085452.

114. Fell DB, Dhinsa T, Alton GD, et al. Association of COVID-19 Vaccination in Pregnancy With Adverse Peripartum Outcomes. JAMA. 19 avr 2022;327(15):1478-87.

115. Jarraya A, Zghal J, Abidi S, et al. Subarachnoid morphine versus TAP blocks for enhanced recovery after caesarean section delivery: A randomized controlled trial. Anaesth Crit Care Pain Med. Déc 2016;35(6):391-3.

116. Qi H, Luo X, Zheng Y, et al. Safe delivery for pregnancies affected by COVID-19. BJOG Int J Obstet Gynaecol. Juill 2020;127(8):927-9.

117. Jarraya A, Choura D, Mejdoub Y, et al. New predictors of difficult intubation in obstetric patients: A prospective observational study. rends in Anaesthesia and Critical Care. 2019;24: 22-25.

118. Sandall J, Tribe RM, Avery L, et al. Shortterm and long-term effects of caesarean section on the health of women and children. Lancet Lond Engl. 13 oct 2018;392(10155):1349-57.

119. Sharma S, Dhakal I. Cesarean vs Vaginal Delivery : An Institutional Experience. JNMA J Nepal Med Assoc. févr 2018;56(209):535-9.

120. Havers FP, Patel K, Whitaker M, et al. Laboratory-Confirmed COVID-19-Associated Hospitalizations Among Adults During SARS-CoV-2 Omicron

BA.2 Variant Predominance - COVID-19-Associated Hospitalization Surveillance Network, 14 States, June 20, 2021-May 31, 2022. MMWR Morb Mortal Wkly Rep. 26 août 2022;71(34):1085-91.

121. Whittaker R, Bråthen Kristofferson A, Valcarcel Salamanca B, et al. Length of hospital stay and risk of intensive care admission and in-hospital death among COVID-19 patients in Norway: a register-based cohort study comparing patients fully vaccinated with an mRNA vaccine to unvaccinated patients. Clin Microbiol Infect Off Publ Eur Soc Clin Microbiol Infect Dis. juin 2022;28(6):871-8.

122. Stock SJ, Carruthers J, Calvert C, et al. SARS-CoV-2 infection and COVID-19 vaccination rates in pregnant women in Scotland. Nat Med. mars 2022;28(3):504-12.

123. Engjom H, van den Akker T, Aabakke A, et al. Severe COVID-19 in pregnancy is almost exclusively limited to unvaccinated women - time for policies to change. Lancet Reg Health Eur. févr 2022;13:100313.

124. Carr EJ, Wu M, Harvey R, et al. Omicron neutralising antibodies after COVID-19 vaccination in haemodialysis patients. Lancet Lond Engl. 2022;399(10327):800-2.

125. Cheng SMS, Mok CKP, Leung YWY, et al. Neutralizing antibodies against the SARS- CoV-2 Omicron variant BA.1 following homologous and heterologous CoronaVac or BNT162b2 vaccination. Nat Med. mars 2022;28(3):486-9.

126. Jarraya A, Kammoun M, Kanoun M, et al. Does COVID-19 vaccination still have a role in maternal and perinatal outcomes during the Omicron era? A multicentre observational study. . Ital J Gynaecol Obstet 2023;35 (4): 433-441. doi: 10.36129/jog.2022.85

127. Chotpitayasunondh T, Fischer TK, Heraud J, et al. Influenza and COVID-19: What does co-existence mean? Influenza Other Respir Viruses. mai 2021;15(3):407-12.

128. **Bolze A, Basler T, White S**, et al. Evidence for SARSCoV-2 Delta and Omicron co- infections and recombination. Med NYN. 9 déc 2022;3(12):848-859.e4.

129. **Popovic M.** Strain wars 3: Differences in infectivity and pathogenicity between Delta and Omicron strains of SARS-CoV-2 can be explained by thermodynamic and kinetic parameters of binding and growth. Microb Risk Anal. déc 2022;22:100217.

130. **Fan Y, Li X, Zhang L, et al.** SARS-CoV-2 Omicron variant: recent progress and future perspectives. Signal Transduct Target Ther. 28 avr 2022;7(1):1-11.

131. **Califano G, Gragnano E.** Life After COVID-19: get your unit ready. Ital J Gynaecol Obstet. sept 2022;35(2):133-135.

132. **Kammoun M, Jarraya A, Ellouze Y, et al.** The impact of COVID-19 booster vaccination in the current pregnancy during the Omicron waves on maternal and perinatal outcomes: a multicentre observational study. . Ital J Gynaecol Obstet. 2023; 35 (4): 550-559. doi: 10.36129/jog.2023.100

133. **Garg I, Shekhar R, Sheikh AB, Pal S**. COVID-19 Vaccine in Pregnant and Lactating Women: A Review of Existing Evidence and Practice Guidelines. Infect Dis Rep. 31 juill 2021;13(3):685-99.

134. **Halasa NB, Olson SM, Staat MA, et al**. Maternal Vaccination and Risk of Hospitalization for Covid-19 among Infants. N Engl J Med. 14 juill 2022;387(2):109-19.

135. **Molloy EJ, Nakra N, Gale C, Dimitriades VR, Lakshminrusimha S.** Multisystem inflammatory syndrome in children (MIS-C) and neonates (MIS-N) associated with COVID- 19: optimizing definition and management. Pediatr Res. mai 2023;93(6):1499- 508.

136. **Piekos SN, Price ND, Hood L, Hadlock JJ.** The impact of maternal SARS-CoV-2 infection and COVID-19 vaccination on maternal-fetal outcomes. Reprod Toxicol Elmsford N. déc 2022;114:33-43.

137. Olearo F, Radmanesh LS, Felber N, et al. Anti- SARS-CoV-2 antibodies in breast milk during lactation after infection or vaccination: A cohort study. J Reprod Immunol. 1 sept 2022;153:103685.

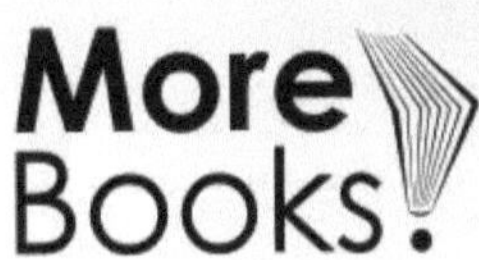

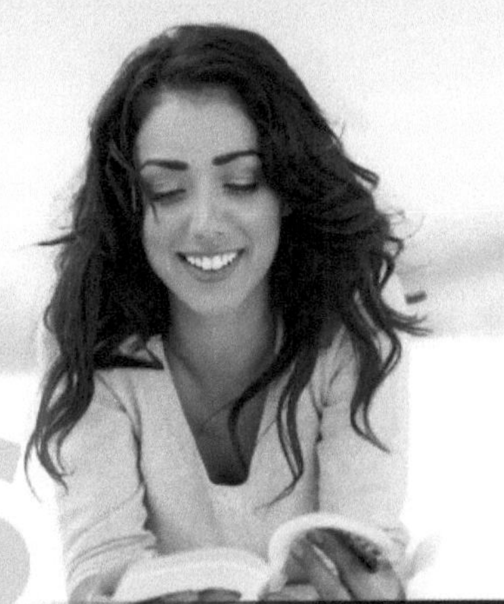

Buy your books fast and straightforward online - at one of world's fastest growing online book stores! Environmentally sound due to Print-on-Demand technologies.

Buy your books online at
www.morebooks.shop

Kaufen Sie Ihre Bücher schnell und unkompliziert online – auf einer der am schnellsten wachsenden Buchhandelsplattformen weltweit! Dank Print-On-Demand umwelt- und ressourcenschonend produziert.

Bücher schneller online kaufen
www.morebooks.shop

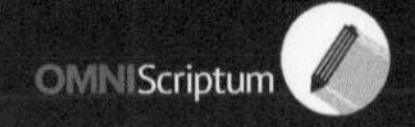

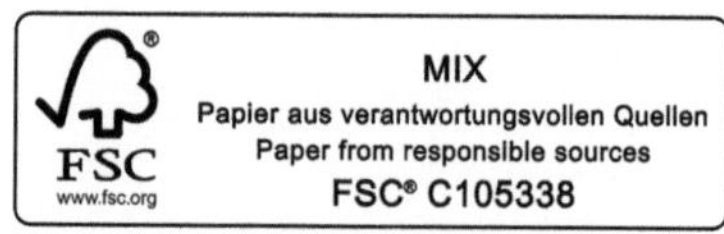

Printed by Books on Demand GmbH, Norderstedt / Germany